Laparoscopic Donor Nephrectomy

Mahesh R. Desai • Arvind P. Ganpule
Editors

Laparoscopic Donor Nephrectomy

A Step-by-Step Guide

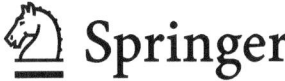 Springer

Editors
Mahesh R. Desai
Department of Urology
Muljibhai Patel Urological Hospital
Nadiad, Gujarat
India

Arvind P. Ganpule
Department of Urology
Muljibhai Patel Urological Hospital
Nadiad, Gujarat
India

ISBN 978-981-10-2847-2   ISBN 978-981-10-2849-6   (eBook)
DOI 10.1007/978-981-10-2849-6

Library of Congress Control Number: 2017936993

Printed on acid-free paper

This Springer imprint is published by Springer Nature
The registered company is Springer Nature Singapore Pte Ltd.
The registered company address is: 152 Beach Road, #21-01/04 Gateway East, Singapore 189721, Singapore

Foreword

This book was an ambitious project, and I suspect it will be the first of many editions. The 13 chapters provide in-depth coverage of the donor evaluation, including financial, emotional, and legal issues, special anesthetic considerations, and the standard techniques of laparoscopic and retroperitoneoscopic donor nephrectomy. Two-thirds of the way through the book, we are teased with descriptions of laparoendoscopic single-site surgery (LESS) and robot-assisted laparoscopic donor nephrectomy procedures and left with the thought that one, or both of them, may be developed into the new standard of care. The final chapter is a visit to the technique of open donor nephrectomy, a procedure that has served us and our patients well for decades.

When considering the adoption of a donor nephrectomy technique, there are common variables to consider: treatment goals (safety for the donor, anatomically useable kidney for the recipient, acceptable kidney function in donor and recipient), financial goals (cost-effective for the healthcare system and the medical center, early return to work for the donor), marketing advantage (for surgeon and medical center), and learning and anxiety curves of the surgical team.

The living renal donor deserves a safe operation, and this book describes how to do it.

John M. Barry, MD
Professor of Urology and Surgery
Division of Abdominal Organ Transplantation
The Oregon Health & Science University
Portland, Oregon
USA

Preface

Primum non nocere which means "first do no harm" aptly describes the principles and practice of donor nephrectomy. The past decade has seen great interest in development of the technique of laparoscopic donor nephrectomy (LDN) across the globe. LDN is a unique operation as the surgeon operates in a pristine milieu on an individual who in fact is not a patient but an individual donating from an altruistic motive. It is also unique as it is a "zero-error" operation because the graft, the donor, and the recipient safety are simultaneously at stake. The procedure is not only of interest to the treating physician such as urologists, general surgeons, and transplant surgeons but also the anesthesiologist and the medical social workers. Laparoscopic donor nephrectomy can be performed via the retroperitoneal or transperitoneal approach. The "new kids" on the block are single-port surgery also known as SILS (single-incision laparoscopic surgery) or LESS (laparoendoscopic single-site surgery). Robot-assisted laparoscopic donor nephrectomy has recently been performed at few centers and is in evolution.

We embarked on this project keeping this in mind and with the intent to emphasize on the technique of LDN. In this volume, we emphasize on the technique of laparoscopic donor nephrectomy in a stepwise manner which includes details of intricacies such as port positioning, steps of dissection, securing the hilum, and retrieval. We focus on the literature support for this procedure. The nontechnical issues which include specifics on donor workup and legal and social aspects will also be dealt in this volume.

The aim of this book is fourfold:

1. Allude to screening and selection of living related donors.
2. Plan a "step-by-step" surgical approach to live donor nephrectomy.
3. Intraoperative management of a living related donor.
4. Understand various approaches to the operation, which include standard laparoscopy, LESS donor nephrectomy, and robotic donor nephrectomy.

A lot of efforts have gone in from all the authors to make sure that the book sees the light of the day. We thank Springer and in particular Mr. Naren Agarwal and Mr. Pandian for making us succeed in this endeavor.

Arvind P. Ganpule
Mahesh R. Desai

Contents

About the Editors

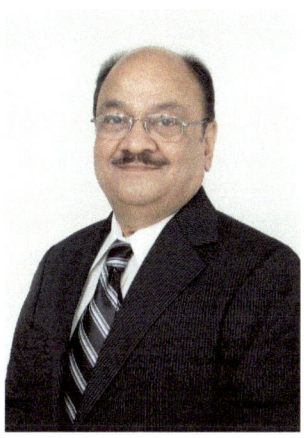

Mahesh R. Desai obtained his MBBS (1966) and MS in general surgery (1970) from B.J. Medical College, Pune University. He received fellowship (FRCS) from the Royal College of Surgeons of London and Edinburgh in 1973 and FACS in 2015. He has held many national and international positions in the field of urology such as president, Urological Society of India (2006–2007); president, Societe Internationale d'Urologie (SIU) (October, 2011–2012); and president, Endourological Society (2012–2013).

Dr. Desai has conducted more than 2500 renal transplants and 900 laparoscopic donor nephrectomies. He has published 150 scientific papers in indexed journals and contributed in more than 30 books. He was awarded the Dr. B.C. Roy National Award for the year 2000 by the President of India. He has also received the President's Gold Medal of the Urological Society of India and American Urological Associations, Presidential Citation for the year 2012, and Life Time Achievement Award from the Endourological Society for the year 2014. He is the recipient of St. Paul's Medal (2012) by the British Association of Urological Surgeons.

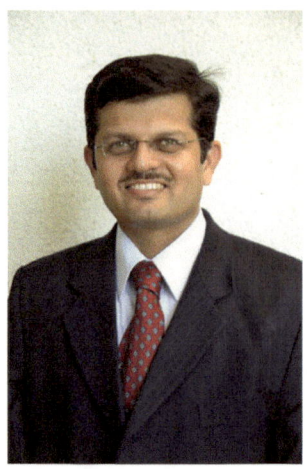

Arvind P. Ganpule is currently vice-chairman in the Department of Urology and chief in the Division of Laparoscopic and Robotic Surgery at Muljibhai Patel Urological Hospital (MPUH), Nadiad, India. He has over 115 publications to his credit in reputed peer-reviewed journals. He has authored a book and 25 book chapters. He was a lead investigator in the largest epidemiological study in India, investigating the natural history of BPH in western India. He has innovated a novel low-cost retrieval bag in laparoscopy known as the Nadiad bag. He was also involved with the team at MPUH, Nadiad, India, in developing the MicroPerc™ system with PolyDiagnost™ GmBH. His area of special interest is laparoscopic approach to donors and robotic kidney surgery.

He is on the editorial board of the *Indian Journal of Urology* (IJU) and *Journal of Minimal Access Surgery* (JMAS). He has been on the editorial board of *SpringerPlus* as well. He was entitled "Best National Reviewer" for the IJU and the Endourological Society (Engineering Section) in the year 2012 and 2015.

Dr. Ganpule is a recipient of the prestigious MIUC scholarship of the Urological Society of India. He has also received the F1000 AFM travel award and grant (for excellent post-publication reviews) consecutively for 3 years (2012–2014). He was entitled the "AUA-USI (Chakravarty fellowship)" scholar for year 2012.

The Evolution of Laparoscopic Donor Nephrectomy: Has It Now Become the Gold Standard?

Sameer M. Deshmukh and Inderbir S. Gill

Abstract

Renal transplantation is the preferred treatment for end stage renal disease (ESRD). Outcomes after transplantation of a kidney from a living donor are superior to those of organs obtained from deceased donors. Traditionally performed by means of an open incision, the last two decades have seen rapid and widespread adoption of laparoscopic donor nephrectomy (LDN), with techniques that continue to evolve and improve. Because LDN delivers donor safety and efficiency, offers excellent allograft function, is preferred by donors, potentially increases the live-donor pool, and since it is now the dominant form of live-donor surgery, a legitimate question can now be asked as to whether or not LDN has become the "gold standard" for living kidney donation.

1.1 Introduction

Renal transplantation is the preferred treatment for end stage renal disease (ESRD). Outcomes after transplantation of a kidney from a living donor are superior to those of organs obtained from deceased donors. Traditionally performed by means of an open incision, the last two decades have seen rapid and widespread adoption of laparoscopic donor nephrectomy (LDN), with techniques that continue to evolve and improve. Because LDN delivers donor safety and efficiency, offers excellent allograft function, is preferred by donors, potentially increases the live-donor pool, and since it is now the dominant form of live-donor surgery, a legitimate question can now be asked as to whether or not LDN has become the "gold standard" for living kidney donation.

S.M. Deshmukh • I.S. Gill (✉)
USC Institute of Urology, Keck School of Medicine, University of Southern California, Los Angeles, CA, USA
e-mail: gillindy@gmail.com

© Springer Nature Singapore Pte Ltd. 2017
M.R. Desai, A.P. Ganpule (eds.), *Laparoscopic Donor Nephrectomy*,
DOI 10.1007/978-981-10-2849-6_1

Donor nephrectomy is a unique surgical procedure because it is performed on a healthy individual who is undergoing the procedure for altruistic motives. Because of this, the operation is truly a high-stakes endeavor with little to no room for error. The safety of the donor, the graft, and the recipient are all paramount and must be taken into consideration when considering any procedural deviation from the standard of care. For the ESRD patient, what is clearly known and documented in the literature are that (1) transplantation is better than dialysis and (2) living-donor organs are preferable to cadaveric organs.

At most centers of excellence worldwide, increasingly, donor nephrectomy is now performed laparoscopically, with traditional (open) donor nephrectomy now performed less commonly. In the United Kingdom, 6% of live-donor nephrectomies were performed laparoscopically in 2000; by 2011, this had increased to 90% [1]. This trend parallels data from the United States, where 49% of living-donor nephrectomies were performed laparoscopically in 2000, which has increased to >95% in 2016. As such, the laparoscopic technique can legitimately lay claim to now becoming the preferred option around the world.

1.2   What Comprises a "Gold Standard" in Medicine?

The term "gold standard" as used today in medicine was taken from its original use in finance. As stated by Jurgen, "a gold standard in its true meaning, derived from the monetary gold standard, merely denotes the best tool available at that time to compare different measures." This term should not be confused with a *golden* standard, as no suggestion is made that the test or procedure being evaluated is perfect; all that is implied is that it is a time-honored alternative that is considered to be the current standard of care or best available test/technique in a given field [2]. Gold-standard tests and procedures are not static, and the gold standard of today will someday be replaced by better and more efficient options in the future. As eloquently stated by Versi: "It is the absolute truth that is never reached; gold standards are constantly challenged and superseded when appropriate" [3].

1.3   History of Donor Nephrectomy for Renal Transplantation

The history of renal transplantation dates back to 1945, when the first cadaveric renal transplantation was performed, followed in 1953 by the first living-related renal transplantation [4].

The first successful living-related donor kidney transplant was performed in identical twins in Boston, Massachusetts, in 1954 [5]. During the subsequent 40-year period (1954–1995), living-donor nephrectomy was performed with the open technique through a large flank incision. Drawbacks of the open technique include but are not limited to postoperative pain requiring analgesic medications, wound complications including flank hernia, and pneumothorax necessitating tube thoracostomy as well as a prolonged hospital stay and time to full recovery.

After this 40-year period, significant developments were made in the 1990s. Clayman performed the first laparoscopic nephrectomy in 1990 [6]. Gill and colleagues were the first to show that laparoscopic donor nephrectomy could be performed in a porcine model [7]. Then, in 1995, Ratner performed the first laparoscopic living-donor nephrectomy in a 40-year-old donor; warm ischemia time (WIT) was less than 5 min and the allograft immediately produced urine, with a recipient serum creatinine of 0.7 mg/dL [8]. Laparoscopic living-donor nephrectomy has evolved and been refined tremendously since that time.

1.4   Kidney Transplant Waiting Lists and the Push to Increase Organ Donation

As of this writing, in 2016, 99,886 candidates are currently on the kidney transplant waiting list, the most of any currently transplanted organ [9]. This waiting list has grown significantly since 2001, when 47,830 patients were waiting for an organ. In 2015, there were 17,878 kidney transplants in the United States, of which 5628 were living-donor transplants. While the number of total kidney transplants continues to increase, the number of living-donor transplants has remained relatively static for at least the last 5 years. Deceased donor transplants outnumbered living-donor transplants by a ratio of 2.5:1 in 2015. This underscores the need to continue efforts to promote living kidney donation, as numerous previous studies have documented the overall quality of a kidney from a live donor is indeed far superior to a cadaveric organ.

Over the past 15 years, during which we have seen an almost doubling of the kidney transplant waiting list, there has also been a significant increase in the proportion of patients older than 50 years of age listed for renal transplantation. Numerous studies over the years have shown that living-donor transplants are associated with better short- and long-term kidney function, as well as with fewer technical graft failures than cadaveric donation. Because of this, over time many different strategies have been employed to increase the number of living kidney donors [10]. These include ABO-incompatible transplants with and without splenectomy, emotionally related donation, cross-over transplantation, genetically unrelated donation, and transplantation of somewhat abnormal kidneys. Laparoscopic donor nephrectomy represents another major effort to increase the overall pool of live donors by making kidney donation and its associated recovery period a more palatable experience for the donor.

1.5   Laparoscopic Donor Nephrectomy Is Being Performed in the Vast Majority of Cases

Laparoscopic donor nephrectomy has been widely adopted since its development, and as a matter of practicality, it is already being performed in the vast majority of living-donor nephrectomies in current times. In a review matching integrated US transplant registry data with administrative records from an academic hospital consortium of 97 centers from 2008 to 2012, the authors identified 14,964 living kidney donations of which 93.8% were performed laparoscopically; of these, 2.4% were performed with robotic assistance, and *only 3.7% were planned open procedures* [11]. In this series, 16.8% of all patients had any complication, but only 2.5% of these complications were Clavien grade 4 or higher. Correlates of Clavien grade 4 or higher complications were African American race, obesity, preexisting hematologic or psychiatric illness, and robotic nephrectomy. Annual center volume higher than 50 cases per year was protective. These data attest to the fact that laparoscopic donor nephrectomy now comprises over 90% of all live-donor nephrectomies at academic medical centers in the modern era.

1.6   Has the Laparoscopic Technique Led to an Increase in the Number of Donors?

Laparoscopic kidney donation has been shown to result in less postoperative pain, quicker recovery, and better cosmetic outcomes. Taken together, these improvements over open surgery (with its associated larger incision) make LDN a more palatable option to the donor, which may lessen some of the disincentives to kidney donation.

Laparoscopic nephrectomy for T1 and T2 renal tumors has been widely accepted as the gold standard for at least 10 years [12]. Whether or not this standard can be applied to living kidney donation has not been widely agreed upon at least to this point. Indeed, even publications as recent as 2010 indicate that "there is no strong evidence that LLDN is better than OLDN" [13]. As such, universal consensus yet remains to be achieved on this issue.

Laparoscopic donor nephrectomy may be more attractive to potential kidney donors, who by definition are otherwise healthy and are altruistically incurring the risks of surgery and anesthesia for the benefit of the organ recipient. As expected, recovery is quicker and postoperative pain lesser in patients undergoing LDN as compared to open surgery. In one study, the duration of postoperative analgesic requirement was 7 days after LDN vs. 30 days after ODN [14]. Additionally, LDN patients required significantly lesser amounts of parenteral analgesics, with LDN patients requiring total morphine doses of 36–88 mg vs. 60–265 mg in ODN patients. Ratner et al. showed that the hospital stay was lesser following LDN at 3.3 vs. 4.7 days in ODN patients, and time to return to work was 11–36 days vs. 39–83 days in the two groups, respectively.

In a randomized study seeking to determine the effects of LDN vs. ODN on health-related quality of life, donors undergoing LDN reported less bodily pain in the first 6 weeks postdonation, and this was associated with an improved mental health component of quality of life compared with ODN (51.9 ± 7.2 vs. 45.3 ± 10.1; $p = 0.0009$) [15].

1.7   What Are the Differences in Postoperative Graft Function Between LDN and ODN?

Ultimately, graft function can be considered the most important factor in determining whether or not laparoscopic live-donor nephrectomy can be considered to have replaced open donor nephrectomy as the "gold-standard" procedure. The first randomized clinical trial comparing these two surgical approaches showed no difference in the serum creatinine level between laparoscopic and open donor nephrectomy grafts at 3 days, 30 days, and 3 months after kidney transplantation [16]. Warm ischemia time was significantly longer in the LDN group (6.6 min vs. 2.09 min), but the long-term graft function was not affected.

At 6 months follow-up, there was no significant difference in the serum creatinine (1.64 mg/dl in the laparoscopic group vs. 1.48 mg/dl in the open group). Laparoscopic and open donor nephrectomies have also been compared in patients with multiple renal arteries, and again postoperative serum creatinine levels and graft survival rates were equivalent [17, 18]. Similarly, postoperative serum creatinine was similar among open, pure laparoscopic, and hand-assisted laparoscopic donor nephrectomies [19]. Overall, regardless of which technique is employed for donor nephrectomy, there is a 5–10% incidence of delayed graft function. However, numerous studies have demonstrated that the laparoscopic approach is not a risk factor for this baseline rate of delayed graft function.

Less is known about long-term graft performance after procurement via the laparoscopic technique. A large study utilized the OPTN database to assess 5532 patients, comprised of 2685 (49%) laparoscopic vs. 2847 (51%) open living-donor renal transplant recipients reported to the Organ Procurement and Transplantation Network between November 1999 and December 2000 [20]. Follow-up data were available through February 2006 (60+ months). At discharge and at 5 years, graft function was similar for both groups; graft survival at 5 years was 79% in the laparoscopic cohort vs. 80% in the open cohort (P = NS). Acute and chronic rejection accounted for 152 laparoscopic (51%) vs. 148 (46%) open graft losses (P = NS). These long-term data are certainly encouraging as LDN has widely overtaken ODN in the number of living-donor nephrectomies performed today.

1.8   Are There Potential Added Risks/Drawbacks of LDN for Donors?

It has been stated that surgeons need the skills used in open live-donor nephrectomy, a fundamental understanding of laparoscopy, and prior experience with laparoscopic partial and radical nephrectomies to perform LDN safely [21]. In multiple studies, the renal warm ischemia time has been shown to be consistently higher in LDN but does not correlate with incidence of delayed graft function, acute rejection, or allograft or recipient survival. As regards potential morbidity to the donor, blood loss and postoperative transfusion requirements have been similar between laparoscopic and open live kidney donation. Operative time for LDN is longer than ODN but decreases with learning curve. The rate of open conversion has ranged from 0 to 13% in several studies [10] with the most common indication being intra-operative bleeding or vascular injury (65%), followed by less common reasons such as difficult exposure, patient obesity, stapler malfunction, and loss of pneumoperitoneum. Several other LDN series have reported far lower rates of open conversion, at 1–2%.

A large retrospective study reviewed 1045 patients who underwent LDN over a 10-year period from 1999 to 2009 [22]. The authors specifically compared outcomes of the first 250 patients (when LDN was offered to a selective group of patients) to the subsequent 795 patients (when LDN was offered to all medically acceptable donors). Overall operative times significantly improved (212 vs. 176 min), overall complication rates did not change (6.4% vs. 5.5%), and major complication rates significantly declined (4.0% vs. 1.4%). Among the last 795 patients, 1 conversion to open surgery and 1 blood transfusion occurred. There was no mortality. Additionally, no differences in overall or major complication rates were seen when cases involving 200 right-sided nephrectomies, 204 donors with complex renal anatomy, and 148 obese donors were analyzed independently. The authors noted that only one planned open donor nephrectomy has been performed at their institution since 2003 (in a donor with a pelvic kidney with complex vasculature), and they indicated that LDN can be offered to all donors, given the presence of an experienced surgical team.

In a meta-analysis assessing the safety of LDN compared to ODN, relevant studies were found by searching Cochrane CENTRAL, PubMed, and EMBASE databases as of October 2011 [23]. Compared with ODN, LDN resulted in a shorter hospital stay (days; mean difference [MD]: -1.27, $p < .00001$), quicker return to work (days; MD: -16.35, $p < .00001$), and less blood loss (ml; MD: -101.23; $p = 0.0001$) without an increase in donor intra- and postoperative complications or compromise of recipient graft function. Hand-assisted laparoscopic donor nephrectomy (HLDN) had a shorter warm ischemia time (minutes) than standard LDN (MD: -1.02, $p < .00001$). However, length of hospital stay significantly favored standard LDN compared with hand-assisted LDN (days; MD: 0.33, $p < .005$), but operative times, intraoperative blood loss, and donor postoperative complications were not significantly different between the two procedures. Finally, donor postoperative quality of life was improved compared to ODN, with both physical functioning and bodily pain scores favoring LDN over ODN.

1.9   What Are the Contraindications to LDN?

Contraindications to LDN are relative and are quite similar to those for most other laparoscopic procedures. These include patients with potentially hostile or frozen peritoneal cavities due to multiple prior surgeries with adhesions. Vascular anomalies are no longer a contraindication to LDN as the procedure has been shown to be safe in this setting in multiple studies [10, 17, 18]. Similarly, obesity is also no longer a contraindication, though any major surgical procedure may carry more risk in the obese patient [24].

Donor age, importantly, is not considered a contraindication to LDN at this time. In a study, donors older than 70 years of age ($n = 28$) were compared with donors less than 55 years of age ($n = 28$) after matching the two groups for sex, date of surgery, BMI, and immunological features [25]. There was no difference in estimated blood loss, operative time, or cold ischemia time. Mean length of hospital stay was also similar, and there were no complications in either group. Early and intermediate recipient serum creatinine levels were similar between the two groups (up to 25 months of follow-up). The authors concluded that LDN can be performed safely in elderly donors without concern for early- or intermediate-term graft function. This could represent another potential avenue to increase the existing donor pool.

1.10   How Has LDN Evolved Since Its Inception in the 1990s?

Since its introduction in 1995, outcomes of LDN have seen tremendous progress and improvement. These include reductions in vascular and ureteric complications. Initial contraindications for laparoscopic live donation are no longer considered to be so; these include right-sided kidney donation, multiple renal arteries, and obesity. Additionally, several studies have shown no difference in blood loss, ureteral complications, cost-effectiveness, graft function, and early rejection. As mentioned, the slightly longer operative time and warm ischemia time seen in LDN have not translated into poorer graft function.

In the initial experiences, the rate of ureteric complications was higher with LDN compared to ODN, but this has improved with refinement of laparoscopic technique. Ratner et al. described a 9.1% incidence of ureteral complications in the first 110 cases, which decreased to 3% in the last 100 cases [17]. In another study comparing 122 LDNs vs. 77 ODNs, ureteral complication rates were similar between the two groups (6.5% vs. 4.1%, respectively; $p = 0.51$) [26].

Data from a large retrospective analysis of prospectively collected data on all consecutive pure LDN surgeries performed at a tertiary academic medical center ($n = 1325$) between March 2000 and October 2013 show several trends over this 13-year period [27]. Over time, LDN was performed on older patients (mean of 35.7 years in 2000 to 41.2 years in 2013 ($p < .001$)), and blood loss decreased over time (75 mL in 2000 to 21.6 mL in 2013) ($p < .001$). However, other variables such as BMI, operative time, and length of stay remained similar over this period. Interestingly, the authors noted that O.R. time, blood loss, surgeon, year of procedure, laterality, BMI, age, and gender did not significantly predict complications. Additionally, there was no significant difference for Clavien complication rates between the early learning period (first 150 cases) and the rest of the series. The authors concluded that with refinements in technique, the overall complication rates for LDN remained low over this time period, despite progressively older patient age.

This group also retrospectively analyzed prospectively collected data for 1204 consecutive LDNs performed from 2000 to 2012 at a single institution [28]. Overall, 8.2% of LDNs experienced complications, and by modified Clavien classification, 74 (5.9%) were grade 1, 13 (1.1%) were grade 2a, 10 (0.8%) were grade 2b, and 2 (0.2%) were grade 2c; there were no grade 3 or 4 complications. Using multivariable regression, the authors found that ≥ 3 renal arteries and late renal vein confluence reached statistical significance and were associated with more complications. They concluded that while not a contraindication to LDN, surgeons should carefully weigh the risks of complex vascular anatomy in their decision to perform LDN.

1.11 Hand-Assisted LDN Versus Pure LDN Versus ODN?

In comparison to pure LDN, the hand-assisted LDN procedure may confer some advantages including shorter total operative time, shorter warm ischemia time, likely due to more rapid graft retrieval. Disadvantages of hand-assisted LDN include delayed recovery of GI function, longer convalescence, and less optimal cosmetic results. El-Galley and colleagues compared hand-assisted LDN with pure LDN, finding no difference in complications, graft function, or early and late recovery [19].

A large review in 2010 identified 57 comparative studies of open, laparoscopic, and hand-assisted laparoscopic donor nephrectomy and their reported outcomes. LDN was superior to ODN in terms of blood loss, pain as measured by analgesic requirement, duration of hospital stay, and convalescence. Postoperative graft function was not significantly different among the three types of donor nephrectomies. The authors concluded that "all three techniques of live-donor nephrectomy are standard of care" [29].

1.12 Robotic LDN Versus Pure LDN?

With recent advances in and more widespread adoption of robotic surgery, live-donor nephrectomy is also being performed robotically in a number of centers worldwide. While large trials comparing robotic donor nephrectomy (RDN) and LDN are lacking, a recent prospective controlled trial randomly assigned 45 kidney donors to RDN and LDN groups in a 1:2 ratio; there were 27 right-sided and 18 left-sided kidneys [30]. Primary endpoints were donor visual analogue scale (VAS) pain scores, analgesic requirement, and hospital stay. Secondary endpoints were donor intra- and postoperative parameters, graft outcomes, and donor surgeon's difficulty scores.

There were no intraoperative complications in either group. VAS pain scores at 6, 24, and 48 h; analgesic requirements; and hospital stay were less in RDN than in LDN. Longer graft arterial length could be preserved with the robotic approach on the right side but not on the left. The RDN group required more number of ports, longer warm ischemia time (WIT), and longer graft retrieval time. Total operative time, hemoglobin drop, postoperative donor complications, and recipient eGFR (estimated glomerular filtration rate) at 9 months were similar in both groups.

The authors concluded that RDN is safe and may be associated with a better morbidity profile than LDN. Clearly, larger trials are needed to confirm these findings, but the study represents an important step in the continued evolution of living-donor nephrectomy surgery.

1.13 What Is the Evidence that LDN Can Now Be Considered the "Gold Standard" for Live Kidney Donation?

In 2011, in the Cochrane Database of Systematic Reviews, the authors searched the online databases CENTRAL (in *The Cochrane Library* 2010, Issue 2), MEDLINE (January 1966 to January 2010), and EMBASE (January 1980 to January 2010) and hand-searched textbooks and reference lists for all randomized controlled trials comparing LDN with ODN [31]. Overall, 6 studies were identified that had randomized 596 live kidney donors to either LDN or ODN. The conversion rate from LDN to ODN ranged from 1.0 to 1.8%. LDN was generally found to be associated with reduced use of pain medication, shorter hospital stay, and faster return to normal physical functioning. LDN had a longer operative time and longer warm ischemia time than ODN (range, 2–17 min), with no associated short-term consequences.

LDN and ODN were similar for perioperative complications, need for reoperation, early graft loss, delayed graft function, acute rejection, ureteric complications, kidney function at 1 year, or graft loss at 1 year. The authors concluded that LDN is associated with less pain than ODN, and that the overall complication rate and profile are similar.

1.14 Cost of LDN Versus ODN

Mullins and colleagues retrospectively compared Medicare expenditures among LDN, ODN, cadaveric renal transplantation, and continued dialysis [32]. They assessed charges for patients with ESRD using both institutional and physician/supplier charges from the United States Renal Data System. Subjects were classified as laparoscopic living-donor transplant, living-donor transplant (open donor nephrectomy), cadaveric transplant, or dialysis patients. Monthly charges were plotted from 12 months before and up to 48 months after the index date (i.e., date of first treatment). There were 230,769 dialysis patients and 44,063 transplant patients (181 laparoscopic living-donor, 11,466 open living-donor, and 32,416 cadaveric renal transplantations). Twelve months prior to the index date, institutional charges were similar between the groups. In the month after the index date, charges were higher for transplantation and then lower in subsequent periods. Two years after the index date, monthly institutional charges were similar for the open living-donor ($191,374) and laparoscopic living-donor ($192,053) transplant patients, followed by the cadaveric transplant ($229,449) and dialysis ($250,348) patients. Physician/supplier charges were highest for laparoscopic living-donor transplant ($104,583), followed by dialysis ($73,730), cadaveric transplant ($70,369), and open living-donor transplant ($65,897). The authors also noted that the break-even points for the open living-donor, laparoscopic living-donor, and cadaveric transplant patients compared with the dialysis patients were 10, 14, and 18 months, respectively.

It is clear that both laparoscopic and open donor nephrectomy confer cost savings over cadaveric transplantation and dialysis [32]. Ultimately, the major determinants of a cost difference between LDN and ODN boil down to the cost of surgical equipment (higher for LDN) vs. the cost of the subsequent hospital stay (higher for ODN). Wolf and colleagues in 2000 showed a higher cost for LDN in their series (overall cost was 73% greater) but after including loss-of-work income due to open surgery and lower hospital costs due to a shorter stay, there was no longer a statistically significant difference in cost ($p = 0.10$) [33]. Clearly, additional studies evaluating costs are necessary, but it seems safe to say that LDN results in higher costs for surgical supplies during the operation, yet results in cost savings due to the reduced hospital stay and the donor's subsequent hastened return to the workforce.

Conclusion

Laparoscopic donor nephrectomy has been widely and rapidly adopted since its inception in the mid-1990s. Surgical outcomes have steadily improved over time, with a dramatic reduction in both vascular and ureteral complications over the past 20 years. As experience has increased, former contraindications to LDN (obesity, age, vascular anomalies, and right-sided donor kidney) no longer exist.

Over 95% of all living-donor nephrectomies in the United States are now performed laparoscopically, and thus it appears as a matter of practicality that LDN has already replaced ODN as the standard of care. LDN is more appealing to potential donors due to less postoperative pain, improved cosmesis, shorter hospital stay, and an overall quicker return to full daily activities and work. LDN and ODN are similar in terms of blood loss, ureteral complications, and early and late graft function. There is also no significant difference in cost-effectiveness between these two techniques. While large, prospective randomized trials with long follow-up are lacking (and will never be done), robust data are already at hand that attest to the wide acceptance of LDN.

Since LDN delivers donor safety and efficiency (decreased morbidity, improved cosmesis, quicker recovery to normal activities), since it delivers excellent allograft function, since it is preferred by donors, since it removes certain disincentives to live renal donation potentially increasing the live-donor pool, and since it is now the dominant form of live-donor surgery comprising approximately 95% of all donor nephrectomies, laparoscopic live-donor nephrectomy has now largely replaced open surgery and assumed the mantle of the "gold-standard" procedure for living kidney donation.

References

1. Banga N, Nicol D. Techniques in laparoscopic donor nephrectomy. BJU Int. 2012;110(9): 1368–73.
2. Claassen JA. The Gold standard: not a golden standard. Br Med J. 2005;330:1121.
3. Versi E. "Gold standard" is an appropriate term. BMJ. 1992;305(6846):187.
4. Smith SL. Tissue and organ transplantation. St. Louis: Mosby Year-book; 1990.
5. Merrill JP, Murray JE, Harrison JH, Guild WR. Successful homotransplantation of the human kidney between identical twins. JAMA. 1956;160(4):277–82.
6. Clayman RV, Kavoussi LR, Soper NJ, Dierks SM, Merety KS, et al. Laparoscopic nephrectomy. N Engl J Med. 1991;324(19):1370–1.
7. Gill IS, Carbone JM, Clayman RV, Fadden PA, Stone MA, et al. Laparoscopic live-donor nephrectomy. J Endourol. 1994;8(2):143–8.
8. Ratner LE, Ciseck LJ, Moore RG, Cigarroa FG, Kaufman HS, et al. Laparoscopic live donor nephrectomy. Transplantation. 1995;60(9):1047–9.
9. UNOS (United Network for Organ Sharing) website. https://www.unos.org/
10. Alston C, Spaliviero M, Gill IS. Laparoscopic donor nephrectomy. Urology. 2005;65(5): 833–9.
11. Lentine KL, Lam NN, Axelrod D, Schnitzler MA, Garg AX, et al. Perioperative complications after living kidney donation: a national study. Am J Transplant. 2016;16(6):1848–57.
12. Raghuram S, Godbole HC, Dasgupta P. Laparoscopic nephrectomy: the new gold standard? Int J Clin Pract. 2005;59(2):128–9.
13. Lechevallier E. Laparoscopic living-donor nephrectomy: is it really better? Eur Urol. 2010;58(4):510–1; discussion 512–3.
14. Ratner LE, Hiller J, Sroka M, Weber R, Sikorsky I, et al. Laparoscopic live donor nephrectomy removes disincentives to live donation. Transplant Proc. 1997;29(8):3402–3.
15. Nicholson ML, Elwell R, Kaushik M, Bagul A, Hosgood SA. Health-related quality of life after living donor nephrectomy: a randomized controlled trial of laparoscopic versus open nephrectomy. Transplantation. 2011;91(4):457–61.
16. Simforoosh N, Bassiri A, Ziaee SA, Tabibi A, Salim NS, et al. Laparoscopic versus open live donor nephrectomy: the first randomized clinical trial. Transplant Proc. 2003;35(7): 2553–4.
17. Ratner LE, Montgomery RA, Kavoussi LR. Laparoscopic live donor nephrectomy a review of the first 5 years. Urol Clin North Am. 2001;28(4):709–19.
18. Gürkan A, Kaçar S, Başak K, Varilsüha C, Karaca C. Do multiple renal arteries restrict laparoscopic donor nephrectomy? Transplant Proc. 2004;36(1):105–7.
19. El-Galley R, Hood N, Young CJ, Deierhoi M, Urban DA. Donor nephrectomy: a comparison of techniques and results of open, hand assisted and full laparoscopic nephrectomy. J Urol. 2004;171(1):40–3.
20. Troppmann C, Perez RV, McBride M. Similar long-term outcomes for laparoscopic versus open live-donor nephrectomy kidney grafts: an OPTN database analysis of 5532 adult recipients. Transplantation. 2008;85(6):916–9.
21. Simforoosh N, Soltani MH, Basiri A, Tabibi A, Gooran S, et al. Evolution of laparoscopic live donor nephrectomy: a single-center experience with 1510 cases over 14 years. J Endourol. 2014;28(1):34–9.
22. Ahearn AJ, Posselt AM, Kang SM, Roberts JP, Freise CE. Experience with laparoscopic donor nephrectomy among more than 1000 cases: low complication rates, despite more challenging cases. Arch Surg. 2011;146(7):859–64.
23. Yuan H, Liu L, Zheng S, Yang L, Pu C, et al. The safety and efficacy of laparoscopic donor nephrectomy for renal transplantation: an updated meta-analysis. Transplant Proc. 2013;45(1):65–76.
24. Marcelino A, Mochtar CA, Wahyudi I, Hamid AR. Obese kidney donors in the laparoscopic living nephrectomy era: how safe? Ann Transplant. 2016;21:297–300.

25. Cavdaroglu O, Gurluler E, Cakır U, Gurkan A, Berber I. Laparascopic donor nephrectomy is safe for extremely old donors and provides a good outcome for their recipients. Transplant Proc. 2015;47(5):1296–8.
26. Lind MY, Hazebroek EJ, Kirkels WJ, Hop WC, Weimar W, et al. Laparoscopic versus open donor nephrectomy: ureteral complications in recipients. Urology. 2004;63(1):36–9; discussion 39–40.
27. Treat EG, Schulam PG, Gritsch HA, Liu CH, Xiong S, et al. Evolution of laparoscopic donor nephrectomy technique and outcomes: a single-center experience with more than 1300 cases. Urology. 2015;85(1):107–12.
28. Hu JC, Liu CH, Treat EG, Ernest A, Veale J, et al. Determinants of laparoscopic donor nephrectomy outcomes. Eur Urol. 2014;65(3):659–64.
29. Greco F, Hoda MR, Alcaraz A, Bachmann A, Hakenberg OW, et al. Laparoscopic living-donor nephrectomy: analysis of the existing literature. Eur Urol. 2010;58(4):498–509.
30. Bhattu AS, Ganpule A, Sabnis RB, Murali V, Mishra S, et al. Robot-assisted laparoscopic donor nephrectomy vs standard laparoscopic donor nephrectomy: a prospective randomized comparative study. J Endourol. 2015;29(12):1334–40.
31. Wilson CH, Sanni A, Rix DA, Soomro NA. Laparoscopic versus open nephrectomy for live kidney donors. Cochrane Database Syst Rev. 2011.
32. Mullins CD, Thomas SK, Pradel FG, Bartlett ST. The economic impact of laparoscopic living-donor nephrectomy on kidney transplantation. Transplantation. 2003;75(9):1505–12.
33. Wolf Jr JS, Marcovich R, Merion RM, Konnak JW. Prospective, case matched comparison of hand assisted laparoscopic and open surgical live donor nephrectomy. J Urol. 2000;163(6):1650–3.

Preoperative General and Urologic Evaluation for Laparoscopic Donor Nephrectomy

Oscar Rodriguez Faba and Alberto Breda

Abstract

Living donor kidney transplantation has become an important alternative to supply the shortage of renal donation. The preparation requires a preoperative general and urologic evaluation of the donor and the recipient including medical, psychosocial and economic aspects. This process involves collaboration between multiple health care professions on the side of the donor and the recipient. A major concern to provide a safe procedure is the long-term impact of having a solitary kidney in terms of risk of developing hypertension, proteinuria, and chronic kidney disease. Recent evidence has demonstrated that survival of kidney donors is similar to that of control subjects who were matched for age, gender, and ethnicity. Overall these findings therefore indicate that the individual and the kidney life span are not adversely affected by kidney donation.

2.1 Introduction

A major concern for living donors is the long-term impact of having a solitary kidney in terms of the attendant risk of developing hypertension, proteinuria, and chronic kidney disease. A recent study that followed 3,700 donors over a 12-year period demonstrated that survival of kidney donors was similar to that of control subjects who were matched for age, gender, and ethnicity. Overall these findings therefore indicate that the individual and the kidney life span are not adversely affected by kidney donation [1].

Different countries have different legal formalities for renal transplantation. In general, careful donor evaluation is necessary to avoid excessive risk in the donor. Donor

O.R. Faba • A. Breda (✉)
Renal Transplant Division, Department of Urology, Fundació Puigvert, Barcelona, Spain
e-mail: albbred@hotmail.com

© Springer Nature Singapore Pte Ltd. 2017   13
M.R. Desai, A.P. Ganpule (eds.), *Laparoscopic Donor Nephrectomy*,
DOI 10.1007/978-981-10-2849-6_2

nephrectomy can be performed by various approaches including traditional open surgery or by more minimally invasive technique such as laparoscopy. Moreover, in terms of long-term function, live donor is better than cadaver transplantation. Living donation seems to be an appropriate alternative to cadaveric donation.

Non-maleficence must be considered a primary objective during living donor evaluation. The screening process should identify potentially acceptable donors, quantify the risk, and on this basis exclude unsuitable donors. A suitable candidate for living donation is usually seen 3 months before the surgery. The team should include a nephrologist, a urologist, a living donor coordinator, and a mental health expert.

2.2 Medical Evaluation Process

The medical evaluation process includes a complete medical history and physical examination, with emphasis on renal disease and family history of renal disease [2]. The process should also include laboratory testing to evaluate renal function and determine immunological compatibility, identification of transmissible infectious diseases, a complete evaluation of renal anatomy with cross-sectional imaging, and assessment of age-adjusted cancer screening [3, 4]. Comorbidities, including hypertension, diabetes, and cardio- and cerebrovascular disease, must be investigated and quantified. Multiple blood pressure readings should be taken and basic laboratory studies performed, including a complete blood count, metabolic and lipid quantification, urinalysis, and coagulation studies. A 24-h urine collection is important for creatinine clearance and proteinuria [5]. Patients with a history of renal stones should undergo metabolic testing for evaluation of risk of developing recurrent calculi. Further evaluation of diabetes in high-risk donors should include oral glucose tolerance testing and hemoglobin A1c measurement.

Assessment of the immunologic compatibility of the donor and the recipient requires determination of the donor and recipient ABO type and performance of a crossmatch to detect the presence of donor-specific antibodies in the recipient. Screening of recipients to determine their panel reactive antibodies and to assign specificities to antibodies, if detected, is routinely performed and is critical for interpreting the results of the crossmatch in equivocal cases or when the autologous crossmatch is positive (Table 2.1).

2.3 Contraindications

General contraindications to living donation are [6] (Table 2.2):

- The presence of vascular disease that precludes the arterial and venous anastomoses required for a technically successful transplant
- Recent or current malignancy
- Chronic illness with short life expectancy
- Active substance abuse
- Active infectious process
- Coronary artery disease
- Psychosocial factors that may hinder future adherence to medical treatment

Table 2.1 Evaluation tests

Laboratory tests (renal function/immunological compatibility)
Blood pressure
24-h urine collection to quantify creatinine clearance and measure proteinuria
Oral glucose tolerance test and HbA$_{1C}$ if indicated
Metabolic workup if previous renal stones
Donor ABO typing
Complete blood count with platelet count and differential
Measurement of transaminases
Lipid profile
Complete coagulation studies
Urinalysis and culture
Electrocardiograph
Chest x-ray
Crossmatch performed
Human leukocyte antigen (HLA) typing of the donor may be done
Clinical history and physical examination
Initial interview with specific focus on renal disease and family history of renal disease
Completion of a detailed health questionnaire
Donor education and completion of evaluation of consent
Detailed history and physical examinations by transplant nephrologists and surgeons
Multiple complete vital signs
Detailed evaluation by mental health expert
Interview with independent living donor advocate
Assessment for transmissible infectious disease
Human immunodeficiency virus, hepatitis B and C
Rapid plasma reagin
Testing for tuberculosis (TB) – TB skin testing or QuantiFERON-TB Gold
Testing for *Strongyloides*, *Trypanosoma cruzi*, and West Nile virus for donors from endemic areas
Evaluation of renal anatomy with cross-sectional imaging
Age-appropriate health screening, including cancer screening
Prostate-specific antigen (recommendations based on donor age and family history)
Gynecologic examination with Papanicolaou smear
Colonoscopy
Mammogram
Pregnancy test if indicated
Echocardiography and cardiac stress testing as indicated
Pulmonary function studies and computed tomography scanning of the chest as indicated

As per guidelines patients with previous malignancies can undergo renal transplantation after a period of 2 years. It is not needed in cases of incidental renal carcinoma, in situ carcinoma, focal neoplasm low-grade bladder cancer, or basal cell skin cancer. A waiting time of more than 2 years is necessary in cases of melanoma, breast cancer, colorectal carcinoma, and uterine carcinoma [7].

Table 2.2 Contraindications

	Absolute	Relative
Age	Less than 18 years	Over 65 years (excluded in many programs)
Substance abuse	Active substance abuse	Abstinence from substance abuse with documented completion of rehabilitation
Hypertension	Multiple agents or high doses of single agents for control End-organ injury Additional strong risk factors for cardiovascular disease	Borderline or control with single agents
Diabetes	Diabetes mellitus	Impaired glucose tolerance
Obesity	Morbid obesity (BMI >35) or obesity (BMI >30) with comorbid conditions	Obesity
Renal disease	Evidence of renal disease, including a reduced creatinine clearance (GFR <80 mL/min), proteinuria (>250 mg), or hematuria	Borderline creatinine clearance, microscopic hematuria
Renal stones	Multiple or recurrent renal calculi of a metabolic condition that predisposes to the recurrence of renal calculi	Single renal stone
Infection	HIV, hepatitis B, hepatitis C	Hepatitis B core antibody
Cancer	Cancer, either current or treated but at significant risk for recurrence	
Cardiovascular disease	Coronary or peripheral vascular disease Valvular heart disease	
Renal anatomic abnormalities	Significant discrepancy in the kidney sizes	Vascular anomalies

2.4 Radiologic Evaluation

The optimal imaging modality remains a matter of debate. Angiography, the classic gold standard for defining renal anatomy, is now rarely used. Currently Computerized Tomography Angiography (CTA) or Magnetic Resonance Angiography (MRA) is used to evaluate the donor kidneys, define vascular anatomy, and assess donors for other abdominal anomalies or pathology [8]. These imaging modalities are particularly important for assessing anatomic variations affecting the renal arteries, veins, or ureters (Fig. 2.1), which are an important consideration in determining the suitability of an individual for living kidney donation. In providing precise information on the anatomy of the renal vasculature and possible variants and diseases prior to surgery, CTA has reduced the risks and complications during and after renal transplantation, improving the likelihood of a successful outcome [10]. MRA is, however, considered equally accurate in defining renal anatomy and detecting incidental findings that may influence the decision about an individual's suitability to be a living kidney donor. While MRA has the advantage of avoiding ionizing radiation and potentially

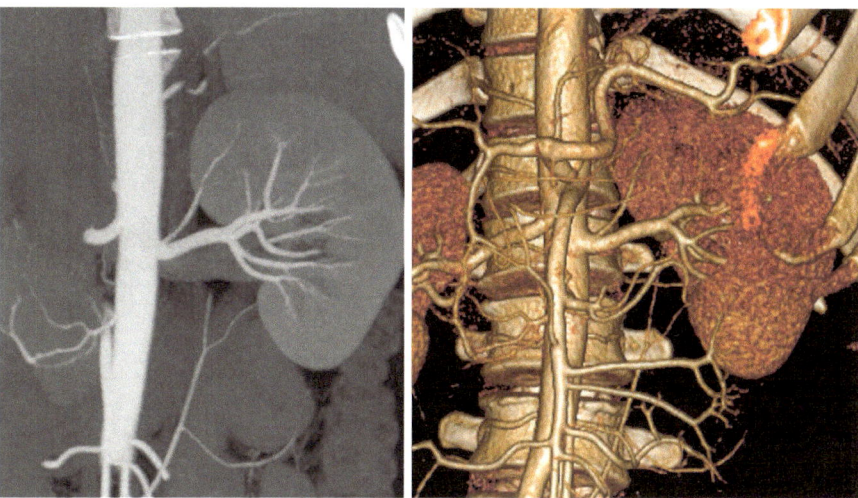

Fig. 2.1 The CTA gives us wealth of information on the arterial anatomy. It gives us an idea about the prehilar branching, the number of vessels, and the relation of splenic vessels to the upper pole

nephrotoxic contrast agents, it is much less sensitive in detecting small renal or ureteral stones [9]. Ultimately the choice of imaging modality should probably be based on local imaging expertise and specific protocols.

All potential donors should have a chest x-ray.

Knowledge of the surgical techniques performed and the exclusion criteria allows radiologists to write an accurate radiological report. The radiological arterial report must include renal artery atherosclerosis, aneurysms, arteriovenous malformations and arteriovenous fistulas, dissection, thrombosis, and fibromuscular dysplasia.

The venous report should include the venous variants of the inferior vena cava (duplication, left location, etc.) and the renal veins (retroaortic, circumaortic) and the location, number, diameter, and variants of gonadal, adrenal, and lumbar veins (Fig. 2.2). A delayed topogram acquired in the excretory phase, delayed CT images, or conventional abdominal radiography must be performed to evaluate the collecting system and ureters and screen for a possible duplication anomaly [11, 12].

2.5 Specific Medical Evaluations

Factors that most commonly contribute to the medical complexity of living kidney donors are age, obesity, hypertension, and psychosocial issues.

2.5.1 Age

There is a clear trend toward accepting older individuals as donors. Registry data indicate that between 2000 and 2009, the mean age of living kidney donors increased

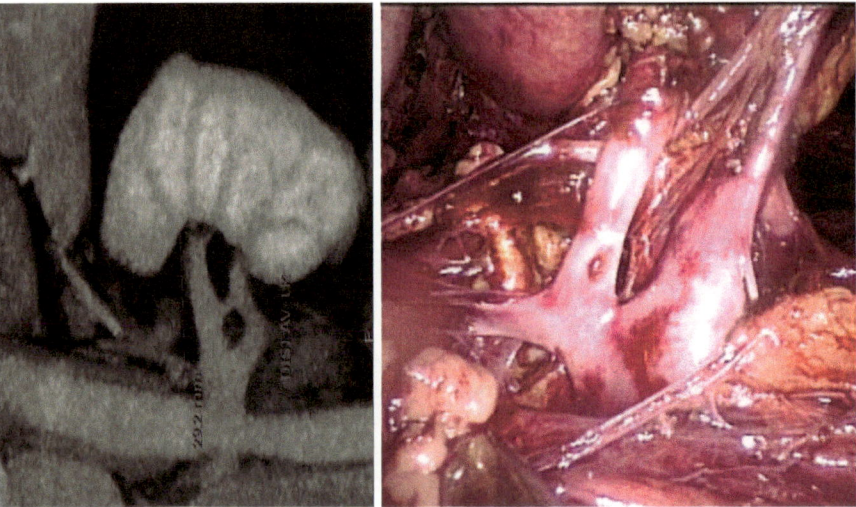

Fig. 2.2 The venous anatomy is also well delineated with the triple-phase contrast CTA. As depicted in this picture the relation of the renal vein with the adrenal vein and the lumbar vein is clearly seen. This is of strategic importance in surgical planning

from 39.6 to 41.3 years, while the percentage of living kidney donors in the 50- to 64-year-old age range increased from 18.1 to 25%, and the percentage of donors between 18 and 34 years of age declined from 33.2 to 30.3% [13]. With respect to the impact of increasing donor age on potential complications, despite the intuitive sense that older living kidney donors might be at increased risk, several groups have reported that the perioperative risk is not increased in older living donors [14, 15].

2.5.2   Obesity

The rationale for excluding obese individuals from living kidney donation has less to do with the technical difficulties related to the surgery or perioperative risk and more to do with the long-term potential risks associated with a unilateral nephrectomy in an obese individual. Extensive data suggest an association between obesity and kidney disease, particularly glomerular diseases. This risk may be increased or accelerated in obese individuals undergoing unilateral nephrectomy for indications other than kidney donation, as reflected by an increase in the prevalence of protein-uria and a declining estimated glomerular filtration rate in individuals with a body mass index (BMI) >30 [16, 17]. Obesity is considered as a risk factor for many diseases including diabetes and hypertension, and IHD's current guidelines have insufficient evidence to exclude patients based on BMI [18].

2.5.3 Hypertension

Traditionally people with history of hypertension were excluded as donors. So not much data is available on long-term outcome of donors with hypertension [19, 20]. Donors should have a blood pressure (BP) of less than 140/90 mm Hg measured on at least three occasions [21].

Donors with evidence of end-organ damage related to hypertension or poor control or other risk factors should be excluded [22].

2.5.4 Psychosocial Issues

The goals of the psychosocial evaluation are to identify behavioral, social, and/or financial issues that may influence compliance and outcomes after transplantation. Proven habitual medical noncompliance or insurmountable psychosocial barriers to posttransplant compliance are a relative contraindication to transplantation. Patients with history of alcohol or any other substance abuse need rehabilitation prior to transplantation. Some centers require patients to abstain from tobacco, particularly when they are known to have cardiovascular disease or to be at high risk (e.g., diabetics). Additionally, some centers consider marijuana use a contraindication to transplantation. Social workers and psychologists trained in the evaluation of transplant candidates perform the psychosocial assessment, with referral for neuropsychiatric assessment if needed. Patients must be able to demonstrate understanding of the potential risks and benefits of transplantation, the need for lifelong immunosuppressive therapy, and the need for compliance with medication and follow-up [23, 24]. Patients with severe cognitive impairment may be acceptable candidates for transplantation, provided that adequate caregiver support and supervised medication administration are guaranteed. Patients with mood, anxiety, or personality disorders should be referred to psychiatry for treatment in order to improve access to and success after transplantation.

2.6 Specific Urologic Evaluations

It is a rule that the best kidney is retained by the donor.

2.6.1 Choice of Kidney

In cases in which both kidneys have similar characteristics, the left kidney is removed since it has the longest renal vein, which facilitates implantation. Right nephrectomy has been associated with more complications, e.g., venous thrombosis, a greater delay in functional recovery, and, in general, a higher incidence of implant loss due to technical difficulties during the vascular anastomosis. Recent studies indicate that in appropriate scenarios, right donor nephrectomy can be undertaken with minimal increased risk [25–27].

2.6.2 Multiple Arteries

The choice of kidneys with multiple arteries has also been a controversial issue. We try to avoid transplantation of such kidneys in order to minimize the vascular and ureteral complications. However, many centers prefer to use the left kidney rather than the right kidney even if the left kidney has multiple arteries. Abnormalities such as circumaortic veins, retroaortic veins, early bifurcation of the renal artery, multiple veins, or large lumbar veins are not usually a problem for the donation. Although all the published studies include only a small number of patients with multiple arteries, globally the transplantation of such kidneys is considered to be feasible and safe. Only in two studies have kidneys with multiple arterial vessels been associated with more ureteral complications in the recipient, the increased risk being especially notable when a kidney with an accessory inferior pole artery is implanted [28–30].

Conclusions

Although much has changed in living kidney donation, the primary goals of ensuring donor health and wellness while still affording recipients the benefit of living donor renal transplantation remain unchanged. The changing health status of the donor population together with the continued evolution of the processes and procedures of living donation provide new challenges that require that the transplant community continually reassess the risks of living kidney donation and develop new policies and procedures to safeguard living donors. Central to the process of minimizing the risk to living kidney donors is the thoroughness of the medical and psychosocial evaluation and the rigor of the process to ensure informed consent by the donor. To this end the donor evaluation process is increasingly complex as the medical, demographic, and psychosocial features of living donors change. Despite these challenges, the careful evaluation of potential living donors continues to provide patients who have end-stage renal disease with the benefits of living donor renal transplantation while simultaneously exposing the donor to low risks.

References

1. Ibrahim HN, Foley R, Tan L, Rogers T, Bailey RF, Guo H, Gross CR, Matas AJ. Long-term consequences of kidney donation. N Engl J Med. 2009;360(5):459–69.
2. Smith RA, Cokkinides V, Brawley OW. Cancer screening in the United States, 2012: a review of current American Cancer Society guidelines and current issues in cancer screening. CA Cancer J Clin. 2012;62(2):129–42.
3. Mandelbrot DA, Pavlakis M, Danovitch GM, Johnson SR, Karp SJ, Khwaja K, Hanto DW, Rodrigue JR. The medical evaluation of living kidney donors: a survey of US transplant centers. Am J Transplant. 2007;7(10):2333–43.
4. Pham PC, Wilkinson AH, Pham PT. Evaluation of the potential living kidney donor. Am J Kidney Dis. 2007;50(6):1043–51.
5. Valapour M, Kahn JP, Bailey RF, Matas AJ. Assessing elements of informed consent among living donors. Clin Transpl. 2011;25(2):185–90.

6. Oikawa M, Hatakeyama S, Narita T, Yamamoto H, Hosogoe S, Imai A, Yoneyama T, Hashimoto Y, Koie T, Fujita T, et al. Safety and effectiveness of marginal donor in living kidney transplantation. Transplant Proc. 2016;48(3):701–5.
7. Penn I. The effect of immunosuppression on pre-existing cancers. Transplantation. 1993;55(4):742–7.
8. Gulati M, Dermendjian H, Gomez AM, Tan N, Margolis DJ, Lu DS, Gritsch HA, Raman SS. 3.0Tesla magnetic resonance angiography (MRA) for comprehensive renal evaluation of living renal donors: pilot study with computerized tomography angiography (CTA) comparison. Clin Imaging. 2016;40(3):370–7.
9. Engelken F, Friedersdorff F, Fuller TF, Magheli A, Budde K, Halleck F, Deger S, Liefeldt L, Hamm B, Giessing M, et al. Pre-operative assessment of living renal transplant donors with state-of-the-art imaging modalities: computed tomography angiography versus magnetic resonance angiography in 118 patients. World J Urol. 2013;31(4):983–90.
10. Chu LC, Sheth S, Segev DL, Montgomery RA, Fishman EK. Role of MDCT angiography in selection and presurgical planning of potential renal donors. AJR Am J Roentgenol. 2012;199(5):1035–41.
11. Holden A, Smith A, Dukes P, Pilmore H, Yasutomi M. Assessment of 100 live potential renal donors for laparoscopic nephrectomy with multi-detector row helical CT. Radiology. 2005;237(3):973–80.
12. Sebastia C, Peri L, Salvador R, Bunesch L, Revuelta I, Alcaraz A, Nicolau C. Multidetector CT of living renal donors: lessons learned from surgeons. Radiographics. 2010;30(7):1875–90.
13. Steel J, Dunlavy A, Friday M, Kingsley K, Brower D, Unruh M, Tan H, Shapiro R, Peltz M, Hardoby M, et al. A national survey of independent living donor advocates: the need for practice guidelines. Am J Transplant. 2012;12(8):2141–9.
14. Balachandran VP, Aull MJ, Charlton M, Afaneh C, Serur D, Leeser DB, Del Pizzo J, Kapur S. Kidneys from older living donors provide excellent intermediate-term outcomes after transplantation. Transplantation. 2012;94(5):499–505.
15. Fahmy LM, Massie AB, Muzaale AD, Bagnasco SM, Orandi BJ, Alejo JL, Boyarsky BJ, Anjum SK, Montgomery RA, Dagher NN, et al. Long-term renal function in living kidney donors who had histological abnormalities at donation. Transplantation. 2016;100(6):1294–8.
16. Praga M, Hernandez E, Herrero JC, Morales E, Revilla Y, Diaz-Gonzalez R, Rodicio JL. Influence of obesity on the appearance of proteinuria and renal insufficiency after unilateral nephrectomy. Kidney Int. 2000;58(5):2111–8.
17. Schold JD, Srinivas TR, Guerra G, Reed AI, Johnson RJ, Weiner ID, Oberbauer R, Harman JS, Hemming AW, Meier-Kriesche HU. A "weight-listing" paradox for candidates of renal transplantation? Am J Transplant. 2007;7(3):550–9.
18. Kalble T, Lucan M, Nicita G, Sells R, Burgos Revilla FJ, Wiesel M. European Association of U: EAU guidelines on renal transplantation. Eur Urol. 2005;47(2):156–66.
19. Ozdemir FN, Guz G, Sezer S, Arat Z, Haberal M. Ambulatory blood pressure monitoring in potential renal transplant donors. Nephrol Dial Transplant. 2000;15(7):1038–40.
20. Meier-Kriesche HU, Schold JD, Srinivas TR, Reed A, Kaplan B. Kidney transplantation halts cardiovascular disease progression in patients with end-stage renal disease. Am J Transplant. 2004;4(10):1662–8.
21. Tent H, Sanders JS, Rook M, Hofker HS, Ploeg RJ, Navis G, van der Heide JJ. Effects of pre-existent hypertension on blood pressure and residual renal function after donor nephrectomy. Transplantation. 2012;93(4):412–7.
22. Young A, Storsley L, Garg AX, Treleaven D, Nguan CY, Cuerden MS, Karpinski M. Health outcomes for living kidney donors with isolated medical abnormalities: a systematic review. Am J Transplant. 2008;8(9):1878–90.
23. Levenson JL, Olbrisch ME. Psychosocial evaluation of organ transplant candidates. A comparative survey of process, criteria, and outcomes in heart, liver, and kidney transplantation. Psychosomatics. 1993;34(4):314–23.
24. Dobbels F, Vanhaecke J, Dupont L, Nevens F, Verleden G, Pirenne J, De Geest S. Pretransplant predictors of posttransplant adherence and clinical outcome: an evidence base for pretransplant psychosocial screening. Transplantation. 2009;87(10):1497–504.

25. Dols LF, Kok NF, Alwayn IP, Tran TC, Weimar W, Ijzermans JN. Laparoscopic donor nephrectomy: a plea for the right-sided approach. Transplantation. 2009;87(5):745–50.
26. Lind MY, Hazebroek EJ, Hop WC, Weimar W, Jaap Bonjer H, IJzermans JN. Right-sided laparoscopic live-donor nephrectomy: is reluctance still justified? Transplantation. 2002;74(7):1045–8.
27. Minnee RC, Bemelman WA, Maartense S, Bemelman FJ, Gouma DJ, Idu MM. Left or right kidney in hand-assisted donor nephrectomy? A randomized controlled trial. Transplantation. 2008;85(2):203–8.
28. Husted TL, Hanaway MJ, Thomas MJ, Woodle ES, Buell JF. Laparoscopic living donor nephrectomy for kidneys with multiple arteries. Transplant Proc. 2005;37(2):629–30.
29. Swartz DE, Cho E, Flowers JL, Dunkin BJ, Ramey JR, Bartlett ST, Jarrell B, Jacobs SC. Laparoscopic right donor nephrectomy: technique and comparison with left nephrectomy. Surg Endosc. 2001;15(12):1390–4.
30. Carter JT, Freise CE, McTaggart RA, Mahanty HD, Kang SM, Chan SH, Feng S, Roberts JP, Posselt AM. Laparoscopic procurement of kidneys with multiple renal arteries is associated with increased ureteral complications in the recipient. Am J Transplant. 2005;5(6):1312–8.

Psychosocial and Legal Issues with Laparoscopic Donor Nephrectomy

3

Sujata Rajapurkar

Abstract

Over the last five decades, kidney transplantation has evolved in both surgical and medical management. The kidney donor faces psychosocial stressors during the decision-making process such as during evaluation, donor nephrectomy, post donation follow-ups, and worries about transplant outcome for recipient and own well-being. This article discusses the psychosocial and legal impact of laparoscopic nephrectomy to help the kidney donor and transplant team to understand better the psychological risk profile and legal requirements of the process of live kidney donation.

3.1   Introduction

Success of live donor kidney transplantation program depends on kidney donor safety. The kidney donor goes through a major surgery performed with altruistic motive. A lot of research and technological advances are constantly focusing on less and less harm to healthy kidney donor and improving their quality of life (QOL) in immediate perioperative period. Quality of life is affected by an individual's physical health, psychological state, personal beliefs, and social benefits [1]. Once selected after extensive investigations, pre- and postoperative care of the donor is of high priority for the kidney transplant management team. Living kidney donation results in significant psychosocial issues for the donor and his family. The psychosocial assessment aims in finding out psychosocial risk factors, such as mental health issues, attitude toward kidney donation, interpersonal relationships among

S. Rajapurkar
Medical Social Work Department, Muljibhai Patel Urological Hospital,
Nadiad, Gujarat, India
e-mail: sujatarajapurkar@yahoo.co.in

© Springer Nature Singapore Pte Ltd. 2017
M.R. Desai, A.P. Ganpule (eds.), *Laparoscopic Donor Nephrectomy*,
DOI 10.1007/978-981-10-2849-6_3

Table 3.1 Kidney donor anxiety scores

	M	SD	t	P
Phase I registration				
Control group	37.2	10.6		
Intervention group	33.4	10.5	1.39	0.08
Phase 2 pre-transplant				
Control group	37.2	10.1		
Intervention group	30.1	10.2	2.72	.004
Phase 3 posttransplant				
Control group	37.1	9.2		
Intervention group	29.8	11.1	2.78	0.003

the significant family member, and concern over body image. Legal issues are specific to each country and may vary from state to state. Transplant teams must adhere to the statutory requirements as specified by their country's legal system.

3.2 Psychosocial Issues

Psychological well-being includes stress, depression, anxiety, emotion, and other psychiatric symptoms. Clemens et al. reviewed 51 English language studies where psychosocial function was assessed using questionnaires in ten or more donors after nephrectomy. Social function included donor's perception of the quality of their personal relationships. Self-concept included donor's feelings of self-esteem and sense of accomplishment. They reported that most kidney donors experience no change or a definite improvement in their psychosocial health after donation [1].

3.2.1 Anxiety

It has been noted that as soon as one comes to know about the need of kidney donation for the survival of a family member, some prospective donors are faced with anxiety, depression, and stresses. A study was conducted to explore the effect of social work counseling on kidney donor anxiety. A structured nephrology social work (NSW) intervention was provided to prospective live kidney donors. Anxiety was measured by a standardized psychological tool, namely, Comprehensive Anxiety Test (CA test). The results suggested that the counseling by a NSW during the kidney donation process lowers donor anxiety [2] as shown in Table 3.1.

Talking about live kidney donation and social worker intervention to discuss with the donors about their self-identified barriers leads to positive results for improved acceptance of the donor and the donor's well-being. Counseling is the most effective form of professional support [3].

In a prospective study, Minz et al. reported that the anxiety trait and state scores were in normal range in postoperative period but were lower than the preoperative scores [4].

3.2.2   Mental Health Checklist and Ability to Donate Out of Free Will

Careful donor selection with appropriate pretransplantation psychiatric consulting allows those with normal life quality to donate without consequence to their physical or psychological status [5]. A mental health specialist should evaluate all prospective donors. Psychosocial evaluation aims in assessing competency, cognitive status, and capacity to comprehend information. The assessment is aimed at removing the risk for exploitation of donors by others for monetary or other gain. It provides knowledge and understanding about donation risks and benefits of surgery, psychological functioning, motivations and expectations, the donor-recipient relationship, social support, and financial stability [6–11]. Majority of transplant programs consider active substance abuse/dependence or active mental health problems or instability to be absolute contraindications to the living donor surgery. Amsterdam Protocol recommends that donors with an alcohol abuse history stop drinking at least 1 month prior to surgery [12]. This should be considered minimum abstinence period, given heavy alcohol abuse can increase postoperative morbidity [13] and risk of acute renal failure [14]. All programs should advise potential donors to quit smoking and chewing tobacco and inform them of their increased risks of cardiovascular disease, cancer, and possible kidney disease [15, 16]. Relative contraindications are history of poor adherence to health care recommendations [6], such donors should be counseled for regular follow-up post donation to monitor health status.

3.2.3   Search for the Kidney Donor

When the patient is told about the diagnosis of end-stage chronic renal failure, many patients due to lack of education are unaware about the intricacies of the procedure. The patient and the family members are explained about his present medical condition and treatment alternatives. The patient and the family members need to have discussions and counseling sessions with the treating doctor and the social worker. If the patient decides to undergo kidney transplantation, then the search for a donor within the family begins. The social worker calls a family meeting of the patient, potential donors, and other decision-making individuals within the family and their spouses. All family members are explained about kidney function and kidney donor selection and rejection criteria. The kidney donors are explained about (i) short-term surgical risks, especially the scar, catheter, and hospitalization; (ii) long-term risk of impaired renal function and hypertension; (iii) loss of time and money; (iv) availability of other treatment alternatives, like maintenance dialysis for the recipient; and (v) the risks and success and failure rates of the transplantation. After understanding these risks, all donors who are deemed suitable are medical worked up.

3.2.4   Decision to Donate

It's the responsibility of the transplant team to know about the decision of kidney donation that it is taken voluntarily and without coercion and pressure from recipient or any other individual. Minz et al. have reported that 4 (5.3%) donors out of 75 donors were under pressure from family or recipient to donate. Two out of them perceived negative impact on health, and one had loss of sleep, and the other was worried about having single kidney [4]. Some transplant programs exercise a "cooling off period" [6] or reflection period to ensure that they have adequate time to consider the information gathered during evaluation process. The allowance of time ensures that the potential donor does not take the decision of donating kidney in haste and has well thought over about the kidney donation. In a study of pediatric transplantations, donors and partners reported an independent decision-making process with no significant influences of partners, relatives, or hospital staff. There was high degree of decision-making process in a live donor kidney transplant (LRKT). Majority of donors did not report negative medical or psychological consequences. The relationship between donor, partners, and recipient child improved after LRKT [17]. A positive psychosocial outcome is encouraged by the following factors: to safeguard against unwarranted coercion, information about realistic expectations to avoid depressive breakdowns, high stability and balanced mutual autonomy in the donor recipient relationship. In addition, information about possible medical and psychological problems helps to prepare for their actual occurrence, awareness of coping strategies and available social support helps to alleviate critical periods after transplantation [18].

3.2.5 Motivational Status

It is noted that strong motivation helps the donor to endure the risk of donation process and plays important role in preventing adverse psychological effect. It is also important to know the motivation for offering to donate out of altruism, love, and affection, as a duty or for any secondary gain. Smith et al. found that 97% of donors reaffirmed their decision about donating kidney, and <15% felt they were pressured to donate [19]. The weight of current evidence indicates that kidney donation has a favorable outcome for both the donor and the recipient, and the participation of living-related donors in kidney transplantation is widely accepted [20].

3.2.6 Ambivalence

Based on a narrative review, it is known that those individuals who are ambivalent about kidney donation are at risk for poor psychosocial outcomes after donation. Intervention is targeted to reduce this risk. Intervention structure and content draw on motivational interviewing principles in order to assist prospective donors to resolve ambivalence. Participants' comments indicated that the intervention addressed their thoughts and concerns about the decisions to donate [21].

3.2.7 Family Dynamics and Relationships

Availability of social support of spouse or other significant family member, friends, and employer is essential to proceed with the kidney donation process. In the event of negative outcome or complication, emotional support from family and friends helps in coping. Whenever there is a search for a kidney donor within the family, it is said that there exists some amount of psychological pressure in some subtle form. In a study by Smith et al. 14.2% of the kidney donors did mention family pressure as one of the reasons for agreeing to donate their kidneys [19]. Among the family members, motivation to donate follows costs and gains factor. The greatest reward is said to be the feeling that you have helped somebody who has been critically ill to restore his life and health. It is noted that in most cases, the donors received a great deal of family praise and gratitude, both before and after for their humanitarian act [22].

The psychological benefit like increase in self-esteem seems to persist even after the allograft (transplanted kidney) has failed. The kidney donation is also reported to improve the relationship with the donor during 12 years period after nephrectomy [19]. The studies of kidney donors have generally shown that they experience long-lasting positive feelings about their decision to donate regardless of the success of transplantation. Many donors are found to report an increased self-esteem and sense of worth. In addition, some donors report an indirect benefit from the improved health of the recipient. Long-term involving follow-up of 20–30 years after kidney donation showed that most donors have high quality of life with a boost in self-esteem and increased sense of well-being.

Living-related kidney donation is associated with generally positive donor-recipient relationship. It is also noted that living-related donors usually demonstrate sustained improved self-esteem and lowered levels of depressive mood posttransplant [23]. In the study of 536 kidney donors done by Smith et al., the relationship between the donor and recipient was described as somewhat or substantially improved after surgery by 13.9% and 28.0% of the donors. If provided an opportunity to reconsider, a majority of the donors stated that they would donate. Their responses were 91.5% definitely, 5.3% probably, 2.9% equivocal, and 0.4% unlikely to donate. These decisions were not related to the success of the graft or the extent of financial hardship created by donation [19].

3.2.8   Body Image

Open surgery was accompanied by long-term complications like mild to moderate incision pain and incisional hernia and a very visible scar leading to diminished body image. In a study, all donors experienced pain, anxiety, and inconvenience during open donor surgery [24]. However, in a study comparing donors who had different operations, the mean body image and cosmetic scores of both laparoscopic and open donors were high and similar [25].

Recently, donor surgery using laparoendoscopic single-site (LESS) donor nephrectomy has been developed for donor comfort and better cosmetics. A randomized comparative study performed at our institute compared postoperative patient pain score and quality of life (QOL) of standard laparoscopic donor nephrectomy (LDN) versus laparoendoscopic single-site (LESS) donor nephrectomy. This study showed that on a select group of donors, LESS patients show early relief of pain with shorter hospital stay with similar complications rate and equivalent graft outcome [26]. Comparative studies with open donor nephrectomy have shown that laparoscopic donor nephrectomy removes some of the disincentives to live donation with shorter hospital stay and faster return to work, without compromising the outcome of the recipient graft function [26].

3.2.9 Marriage and Kidney Donation

The strength of marriage is the mutual trust and understanding between the spouses. It is believed that illness in the family may cause stress on partners which may have an adverse effect on marriage. Kidney donation may add additional stress to already troubled marriages (especially if the donor's spouse is opposed to the donation) [23]. Smith et al. (1986) have noted that out of 371 donors, 27 (7.1%) were divorced or separated at the time of follow-up, and 12 (44.4%) of these reported a failed marriage within 1 year of donation. It is noted that a failed marriage occurred among the donors who were pressurized to donate by other family members [19]. The donors who were married and older than 51 years old had higher scores for posttraumatic growth (PTG) than donors who were not married or younger [27]. In my opinion based on counseling kidney donor families both pre- and postoperatively in over 2,500 cases, I did not find any major marital discord postoperatively. This is probably a result of sociocultural factors, extensive preoperative counseling and taking informed consent of the donor's spouse.

3.2.10 Impact on Employment, Finances

Kidney donation may impact on employment; an important concern is whether the employer will grant leave from work till the donor is completely recovered. Will the donor receive pay during investigations, operation, and post donation recovery period? It is important that the employer has knowledge and understanding about kidney donation. More significant factor being under what circumstances he/she is donating kidney. The employer's positive attitude will help during the convalescence and periodic check-ups lifelong. The support of employer is crucial in lessening financial burden if any. Laparoscopic donor nephrectomy gives kidney donor added advantage of less hospitalisations resuming normal activities and start of work sooner.

3.2.11 Special Issues Like Childbearing

Female donors will be advised to postpone carrying a baby (pregnancy) for a short time and in future if planning to have a child, she should be in touch with a consultant nephrologist to assess the kidney function, during the course of pregnancy. Najarian et al. found donors to be perfectly normal; several had undergone normal pregnancies after donation [28].

Post donation information and discussion with the kidney donor and his family members about several day-to-day activities such as exercise resumption and having normal sexual activity is necessary. The counseling is directed to alleviate fear and to encourage additional lifestyle modifications for better health, such as regular physical exercise, hobby pursuits, and the incorporation of meditation or prayer. Such counseling leads to improvement in total well-being.

3.2.12 Follow-Up

Smith et al. suggested that the relationship developed by the team with the donor rather than the instruments is the major factor in successfully addressing the psychosocial issues [32]. Andersen et al. performed the largest randomized quality of life study by assigning 122 donors to laparoscopic or open surgery. The first reports of this study evaluated donor safety, postoperative pain, and convalescence and concluded that minor benefits at 12 months were hard to prove [30]. A further study by the same group of the donor's subjective assessment and research performed long-term comparison of health status and overall quality of life at 1, 6, and 12 months after surgery. There were no long-term differences in SF-36 scores between the groups [30]. The Heidelberg consultation has proven useful for allowing open discussion about critical issues. Psychological support after transplantation seems to be indicated for monitoring with typical first-year problems [33]. Clinicians should look for possible psychological problems after donation and guide the tailoring of individual psychological interventions. In a study by Langenbach et al., they interviewed kidney donors to investigate the QOL of renal donors and their subjective evaluation of the donation during long-term follow-up. The interviews were audiotaped, transcribed, and analyzed. Three main ideal types of donors were differentiated: the "happy helper," the "ambivalent partner," and the "hypochondriacal complainer." The kidney donors wished for extended counseling after kidney donation [33]. Only a minority of living kidney donors suffer psychosocial morbidity. Better preparation for surgery and mere consistent follow-up could decrease negative outcome further [34]. In living-related women kidney donors, quality of life (QOL) improves, and depression scores decline after kidney donation [35]. Living-related kidney donations did not affect the lives and psychological aspects of donors. Screening donors strictly, perfecting the medical care systems, intensifying follow-up and social support, and providing necessary psychological counseling should be fundamental prerequisites [36]. LDN has several short-term benefits, including a shorter hospital stay and a better quality of life at 1 month postoperatively and may be advocated for these reasons; however, long-term results on physical and psychological outcome are comparable between invasive muscle splitting and laparoscopic approach [29]. In another study by Perry et al., laparoscopy group had significantly less postoperative pain and required less time to return to normal functional activities than invasive muscle splitting group, showing higher quality of life scores [31].

3.3   Legal Issues

In India, each living donor must also receive a thorough psychosocial assessment. These assessments can identify the psychosocial barriers to living donation, and the transplant teams can work with potential kidney donors to ameliorate such barriers. The Human Organ Transplantation Act 1994 stipulates hospitals registered for organ transplant/retrieval to appoint a transplant coordinator who is either a graduate in any recognized medical system or a nurse or a master in social work/psychology/public health and is qualified counselor and can encourage the next of kin of the deceased person to donate human organs and coordinate the process of transplantation. Schover et al. and Russel et al. have suggested that a transplant program should include a mental health professional who advocates safety of donors without being influenced by the plight of recipients [35].

3.3.1   Informed Consent Process

Transplant programs have documented consent process prior to donor surgery. Information about the evaluation, surgery risks, complications, and the follow-up care are commonly reported elements in the consent process; kidney donor should be aware that alternative treatments are available for the recipient [6]. Potential donors should also be made aware of the possible negative psychosocial outcomes reported in the previous literature, experiences including strain in family relationships, impaired body image, depression and anxiety. Informed consent process should include education tailored to kidney donor's level of health literacy and to be provided with additional materials to take home with them to review and discuss with their family members [37].

In addition, novel programs now facilitate the exchange of kidneys among incompatible donor-recipient pairs with excellent outcomes. Each transplant center is required to fulfill the legal procedures mandatory to be followed.

Information about the evaluation, surgery risks and complications, and follow-up care is the most commonly reported in the consent process.

3.3.2   The Human Organ Transplantation Act, 1994 (THOA-94)

The Government of India adopted The Human Organ Transplantation Act in 1994 [38]. Each state has different set of rules and regulations to implement it. The gist of the law essentially is there should be no commercial dealings between the treating professional and also between recipient and kidney donors. The act has defined near-related donors; in 2011 paternal and maternal grandparents were included. It is the responsibility of the treating doctor to confirm the identity of the donor and recipient as well as their relationship. These facts and the informed consents have to be recorded in specific forms to be filled and countersigned by the head of the institution and have to be submitted to local- or state-based authorization committees.

The Appropriate Authority in each state is responsible for forming rules and procedures to be followed by transplant centers and to oversee all transplant activity in the state. Each Hospital Based Authorization Committee (HBAC) should consist of persons of high integrity, social status, and credibility or self-employed professionals like lawyers, chartered accountants, doctors, readers or professors, and renowned well-reputed personalities to be the members of this committee. The committee should have adequate representation of women. It should not have employees of the hospital where the transplant is to be performed. The recipient-donor pair along with their next of kin is to be interviewed by the HBAC for the approval of the transplant. The committee checks the complete forms as stipulated by the act, verifies the identity proofs, and satisfies the no pressure, voluntary consent by the donor without financial transaction between recipient and kidney donor. The HBAC gives approval to the transplant team to do the transplantation. In cases where donor is not a near relative or a paired/swap/exchange transplant after interviewing and verifying the documents, the committee passes the resolution which is signed by two members of HBAC and countersigned by the chairman of HBAC and forwarded to the State Appropriate Authority for the final approval. Foreign national's legal document file is sent to the respective embassy for "No Objection Certificate" (NOC); after receiving the NOC, the file is sent to the chairman of the State Appropriate Authority. The Appropriate Authority schedules the personal interview of the recipient, donor, and next of kin and gives the permission to undertake the transplant. In India some state Appropriate Authorities do not call foreign nationals for personal interview of recipient and kidney donor along with next of kin. In these cases form no. 21, sent by the respective embassy is considered valid for approval.

National Organ and Tissue Transplant Organization (NOTTO) is a national-level organization set up under Directorate General of Health Services and Ministry of Health and Family Welfare, Government of India. On 15 June 2015, all transplant centers were notified that as per THOA rules every hospital doing transplant/retrieval of organ/tissue must be registered with the NOTTO, which is located in New Delhi. Manual regarding registration is available on NOTTO website, i.e., www.notto.nic.in.

3.4   Summary

Every kidney transplant team's prime focus is the kidney donor and donor evaluation; informed consent and ethical consideration are significant. Donors must be given accurate expectations about postoperative recovery. Every kidney donor should receive strong compassionate support during evaluation and pre-, and postoperative period by interdisciplinary team members. The special role of donors is to be acknowledged by the transplant team on an ongoing basis [35]. The areas of concern such as hospital stay, out-of-pocket expenses, potential scarring, risk of immediate complication from procedures, and risk of kidney failure in the future are of foremost importance for the well-being of the kidney donor. Whenever a situation of adverse recipient outcome is noticed at any time frame early intervention and counseling should be facilitated [39]. Kidney donors should have access to meet counsellor for psychological support & counseling services. All efforts are to be directed to prevent a negative quality of life post kidney donation.

References

1. Clemens KK, Thiessen-Philbrook H, Parikh CR, et al. Psychosocial health of living donors: a systematic review. Am J Transplant. 2006;6:2965–77.
2. Rajapurkar S, Browne T, Savage TE. Can a social work intervention reduce kidney donor anxiety? A pilot test. Natl Kidney Found J Nephrol Soc Work. 2013;37:37.
3. DePasquale N, Hill-Briggs F, Darrell L, Boyer LL, Ephraim P, Boulware LE. Feasibility and acceptability of the TALK social worker intervention to improve live kidney transplantation. Health Soc Work. 2012;37(4):234–49.
4. Minz M, Udgiri N, Sharma A, Heer MK, Kahyap R, Nehra R, Sakhuja V. Prospective psychosocial evaluation of related kidney donors: Indian perspective. Transplant Proc. 2005;37: 2001–3.
5. Virzi A, Signorelli MS, Veroux M, et al. Depression and quality of life in living related renal transplantation. Transplant Proc. 2007;39(6):1791–3.
6. Rodrigue JR, Pavlakis M, Danovitch GM, Johnson SR, Karp SJ, Khwaja K, Hanto DW, Mandelbrot DA. Evaluating living kidney donors- relationship types, psychosocial criteria and consent processes at US transplant programs. Am J Transplant. 2007;7:2326–32.
7. Dew MA, Jacobs C, Jowsey S, et al. Guidelines for the psychosocial evaluation of living unrelated kidney donors in the United States. Am J Transplant. 2007;7:1047–54.
8. United States Department of Health and Human Services, Centers for Medicare and Medicaid Services. Requirements of approval and re-approval of transplant centers to perform organ transplants; final rule. Fed Regist. 2007;72:15198–280.
9. Olbrisch ME, Benedict SM, Haller DL, Levenson JL. Psychosocial assessment of living organ donors: clinical and ethical consideration. Prog Transplant. 2001;11:40–9.
10. Leo RJ, Smith BA, Mori DL. Guidelines for conducting a psychiatric evaluation of the unrelated kidney donors. Psychosomatics. 2003;44:452–60.
11. Rodrigue JR, Bonk V, Jackson S. Psychological consideration of living organ donation. In: Rodrigue JR, editor. Bio-psychosocial Perspectives on Transplantation. New York: Kluwer Academic/Plenum Publishers; 2001. p. 59–70.
12. International Forum on the Care of the Live Kidney Donor. A report of the Amsterdam forum on the care of the live kidney donor: Ddta and medical guidelines. Transplantation. 2005;79:S53–66.
13. Tonnesen H, Petersen KR, Hojgaard L, et al. Postoperative morbidity among symptom-free alcohol misusers. Lancet. 1992;340:334–7.
14. Vamvakas S, Teschner M, Bahner U, Heidland A. Alcohol abuse: potential role in electrolyte disturbances and kidney diseases. Clin Nephrol. 1998;49:205–13.
15. Tozawa M, Iseki K, Iseki C, et al. Influence of smoking and obesity on the development of proteinuria. Kidney Int. 2002;62:956–62.
16. Hunt JD, Van Der Hel OL, McMillan GP, Boffetta P, Brennan P. Renal cell carcinoma in relation of cigarette smoking: meta-analysis of 24 studies. Renal cell carcinoma in relation of cigarette smoking: meta-analysis of 24 studies. Int J Cancer. 2005;114:101–8.
17. Neuhaus TJ, Wartmann M, Weber M, Landolt MA, Laube GF, Kemper MJ. Psychosocial impact of living-related kidney transplantation on donors and partners. Pediatr Nephrol. 2005;20(2):205–9.
18. Schweitzer J, Seidel-Wiesel M, Verres R, Wiesel M, et al. Psychological consultation before living kidney donation: finding out and handling problem cases. Transplantation. 2003;76(10):1464–70.

19. Smith, Kappell, Province, et al. Living related kidney donors: a multicentre study of donor education, socioeconomic adjustment and rehabilitation. Am J Kidney Dis. 1986;8(4):223–33.
20. Surman OS. Psychiatric aspects of organ transplantation. Am J Psychiatr. 1989;146:972–82.
21. Dew MA, Zuckoff A, DiMartini AF, DeVito DAJ, McNulty ML, Fox KR, Switzer GE, Humar A, Tan HP. Prevention of poor psychosocial outcomes in living organ donors: from description to theory-driven intervention development and initial feasibility testing. Prog Transplant. 2012;22(3):280–92.
22. Simmons RG. Long term reaction of renal recipients and donors: psychological problem in kidney failure and their treatment, vol. 1. New York: Plenum Publishing Corporation; 1981. p. 227–45.
23. Wolcott DL, Norquist. Psychiatric aspects of kidney transplantation. In: Donovitch GM, editor. Handbook of kidney transplantation. Boston: Little, Brown & Company; 1992. p. 339–55.
24. Taghavi R. The complications and morbidity of flank incision for living renal donor. Transplant Proc. 2001;33:2638–9.
25. Lind MY, Hop WC, Weimar W, IJzermans JN, et al. Body image after laparoscopic or open donor nephrectomy. Surg Endosc. 2004;18:2376–1279.
26. Kurien A, Rajapurkar S, Sinha L, et al. Standard laparoscopic donor nephrectomy versus laparoscopic single-site donor nephrectomy: a randomized comparative study. J Endourol. 2011; 25(3):365–70.
27. YucetinL Bozoklar CA, Yanik O, Tekin S, Tuncer M, Demirbas A. An investigation of post-traumatic growth experiences among living kidney donors. Transplant Proc. 2015;47(5): 1287–90.
28. Najarian JS. Living donor kidney transplants: personal reflections. Transplant Proc. 2005; 37(9):3592–4.
29. Kok NF, Alwayn IP, Tran KT, et al. Psychosocial and physical impairment after mini-incision open and laparoscopic donor nephrectomy: a prospective study. Transplantation. 2006;82(10):1291–7.
30. Andersen MH, Mathisen L, Veenstra M, Oyen O, Edwin B, Digernes R, Kvarstein G, Tonnessen TI, Wahl AK, Hanestad BR, Fosse E. Quality of life after randomization to laparoscopic versus open living donor nephrectomy: long-term follow-up. Transplantation. 2007;84:1.
31. Perry KT, SJ Freedland, Hu JC, Phelan MW, Kristo B, Gritsch AH, Rajfer J, Schulam PG. J Urol. 2003;169:2018–21.
32. Smith GC, Thomas T, Kerr PG, Chadban SJ. Prospective psychosocial monitoring of living kidney donors using the short form-36 health survey: result at 12 months. Transplantation. 2004;78:9.
33. Langenbach M, Stippel A, Stippel D. Kidney donors' quality of life and subjective evaluation at 2 years after donation. Transplant Proc. 2009;41(6):2512–4.
34. Schover LR, Streem SB, Boparai N, Duriak K, Novick AC. The psychosocial impact of donating a kidney: long-term follow-up from a urology based center. J Urol. 1997;157(5):1596–601.
35. Guleria S, Reddy VS, Bora GS, et al. The quality of life of women volunteering as live related kidney donors in India. Natl Med J India. 2011;24(6):342–4.
36. Zheng XY, Han S, Wang LM, Zhu YH, Zeng L, Zhou MS. Quality of life and psychology after living-related kidney transplantation from donors and recipients in China. Transplant Proc. 2014;46(10):3426–30.
37. Parekh AM, Gorden EJ, Garg AX, Waterman AD, Kulkarni S, Parikh CR. Living kidney donor informed consent practices vary between US and non-US centers. Nephrol Dial Transplant 2008;23:3319.
38. Ministry of Law, Justice, and Company Affairs. 1994. The transplantation of human organ act, 1994, no. 42 of 1994. Retrieved from http://www.archive.india.gov.in/allimpfrms/allacts/2606. pdf.
39. Boulware LE, Ratner LE, Sosa JA, Alexander HTu, Nagula S, Simpkins CE, Durant RW, Powe NR. The general public's concerns about clinical risk in live kidney donation. Am J Transplant. 2002;2:186–93.

Anaesthesia Concerns for Laparoscopic Donor Nephrectomy

4

Dinesh Prajapati, Deepak Mistry, Manoj Patel, and Ankush Jairath

Abstract

Anesthesia during laparoscopic donor nephrectomy remains the key component for success. The various aspects that the treating medical professionals should know in this regard are the details regarding the preanaethesia check up, intra-operative management anaethesia related issues and the post-operative care. In this chapter these points are detailed.

4.1 Introduction

Kidney disease is recognized as a major health problem worldwide. There is a long waiting list for renal transplantation. However, the gap between the organ supply and demand has increased. The majority of chronic kidney disease (CKD) patients have to depend on the live-related kidney donor. Live-related donor is the potential source of organs for transplantation at an earlier stage of disease with minimal delay. The graft survival rate is higher in the live-related allograft recipient as compared to recipients of cadaveric donor graft [1–4].

D. Prajapati DA, DNB (Anaesthesia) (✉) • D. Mistry • M. Patel
Department of Anaesthesia, Muljibhai Patel Urological Hospital,
Dr Virendra Desai Road, Nadiad, Gujarat, India
e-mail: dr_djp2011@hotmail.com

A. Jairath
Department of Urology, Muljibhai Patel Urological Hospital,
Dr Virendra Desai Road, Nadiad, Gujarat, India

© Springer Nature Singapore Pte Ltd. 2017
M.R. Desai, A.P. Ganpule (eds.), *Laparoscopic Donor Nephrectomy*,
DOI 10.1007/978-981-10-2849-6_4

35

Previously, donor nephrectomy was done by the traditional approach through a subcostal lateral incision, but it was completely replaced by a laparoscopic approach in last few decades. Melcher and colleagues reported 500 consecutive laparoscopic donor nephrectomies without the need to open or reoperate for technical difficulties [5]. The laparoscopic approach has its own advantages like decreased postoperative pain, reduced hospital stay, early recovery and good cosmetic results [6, 7].

4.2   Preoperative Assessment of Live-Related Kidney Donor

This has been discussed separately by other authors.

4.3   Intraoperative effects of laparoscopic donor nephrectomy

Intraoperative changes during laparoscopy are due to mechanical effect of pneumoperitoneum, position and absorption of CO_2. Pneumoperitoneum raises intra- abdominal pressure (IAP). Physiological changes are minimized if the intra-abdominal pressure is <15 mmHg. This value is monitored on insufflation's equipment [8].

4.3.1   Physiological Effects Due to CO_2 Pneumoperitoneum

(a) *Respiratory changes*: Pneumoperitoneum can lead to upward diaphragmatic displacement, reduce lung volume and compliance, increase airway resistance, increase ventilation/perfusion (V/Q) mismatch, cause hypoxia/hypercarbia and increase risk of regurgitation. Increase in minute ventilation by 15–25 % offsets this problem. If surgery is prolonged, it is advisable to do arterial blood gas analysis to know the acidosis status of the patient [9–13].

(b) *Cardiovascular changes* [8, 14–18]: Pneumoperitoneum can show biphasic changes in cardiac output, increased systemic vascular resistance, raised mean arterial pressure (MAP), compression of IVC and reduced venous return. To maintain the haemodynamic stability, patient should be preloaded with crystalloid fluid before pneumoperitoneum, and creation of pneumoperitoneum should be gradual. During creation of pneumoperitoneum, it leads to increase vagal tone, bradycardia and hypotension, which can be treated by injection atropine.

(c) Renal effects [8, 19]: Pneumoperitoneum is also responsible for the reduction of renal blood flow, reduced glomerular filtration rate and reduced urine output. These are the unfavourable effects for the donor kidney. To counteract these effects, it is always better to keep MAP >100 mmHg and administer diuretics just prior to onset of pneumoperitoneum (intravenous injection of 10 mg frusemide). Urine output monitoring is also required every half hourly to monitor the effect of pneumoperitoneum on renal function.

(d) The other effects of pneumoperitoneum are decreased mesenteric circulation, increased intracranial pressure, increased intraocular pressure [20] and fall in body temperature and should be taken into consideration.

(e) Decreased venous return from lower limbs, decreased venous peak flow rate in the femoral vein, increased femoral venous pressure and reduced venous pulsatility contribute to the development of venous thromboembolism (VTE) and deep-vein thrombosis (DVT). For all indications and all ages, reported incidence of DVT is 50 per 100,000 patients. The incidence of DVT rarely occurs before 20 years, but the incidence increases with age. The incidence of DVT, in patients over 70 years, is 200 per 100,000 [21]. For urological laparoscopic procedures, postoperative VTE has been reported in 0.13–1.3 % [22, 23]. DVT and VTE are important preventable complications that put the patients at risk of pulmonary embolism, recurrent VTE and post-thrombotic syndrome [24]. Usually, urological laparoscopic surgery carries the minimal risk of VTE as per available data on literature. Among the many risk factors, age over-exceeding 40 years, previous VTE, obesity, varices and oestrogen use are especially relevant for surgical patients. Recently, the approach to the problem has become increasingly evidence-based, and some relevant medical professional societies worldwide have recommendation and clinical practice guidelines. According to their recommendation, there are four levels of risk emerged, and preventive strategies need to be applied [25]. As a policy, we ensure that early mobilization, compression elastic stocking and sometimes low molecular weight heparin (LMWH) are the main tools for DVT prophylaxis.

4.3.2 Patient Positioning

Chapter on laproscopic left donor nephrectomy (Chap. 5) and open Donor nephrectomy (Chap. 13) describe the patient positioning.

4.4 Anaesthesia Management

Communication between all concerned (urologist, nephrologist and anaesthetist) is paramount.

Our aim during anaesthesia is to maintain normocapnia, to prevent the haemodynamic and stress response due to pneumoperitoneum, to maintain adequate renal perfusion and urine output and finally to prevent postoperative complications.

4.4.1 Preoperative Anaesthetic Preparation

The donor is admitted 1 day prior to the procedure. An informed and written consent is obtained. The night prior, intravenous cannulation is done for intravenous fluid, primarily crystalloids (normal saline (NS) or ringer lactate (RL)). They are started at an infusion rate of 100 ml/hr during NBM hours. We start maintenance fluid, which will continue until we shift to the operation theatre. The donor is nil by mouth for at least 6–8 h. We give antibiotics and premedication half an hour before shifting in operating room.

Intravenous injection of 4 mcg/kg glycopyrrolate and 0.10 mg/kg ondansetron and intramuscular injection of 30 mg pentazocine are given 30 min prior to induction.

4.4.2 Intraoperative Management

- Monitoring:
  The temperature, electrocardiogram, pulse oximetry, noninvasive blood pressure monitor, end-tidal carbon dioxide and peripheral nerve stimulator are recommended modalities of monitoring. Invasive monitoring like central venous pressure and invasive blood pressure are optional and not required in all cases.
  Adequacy of ventilation during laparoscopic surgery is most commonly assessed by end-tidal carbon dioxide monitoring as a noninvasive substitute for partial pressure of carbon dioxide ($PaCO_2$) in arterial blood.
  An airway pressure monitor, present on the ventilator of anaesthesia machine, is routinely used during intermittent positive-pressure ventilation. An activated high airway pressure alarm can aid detection of excessive elevation in IAP [26]. The use of a Bispectral Index monitor, a possible monitor of the depth of anaesthesia, can help to reduce the occurrence of awareness. It can further assist in titrate intravenous and inhalation agents to fasten emergence and improved recovery [27, 28].
- General anaesthesia with balanced anaesthesia technique, including inhalation agents, intravenous induction agents and a variety of muscle relaxant, is the choice of anaesthesia.
- General anaesthesia with endotracheal intubation is the recommended approach to protect against pulmonary aspiration, aid ventilation and allow IPPV. IPPV is to overcome the respiratory effects of pneumoperitoneum and hypercarbia. Good muscle relaxation reduces the intra-abdominal pressure needed for adequate surgical exposure.
- During preoxygenation: Excess stomach inflation from mask ventilation is to be avoided.
- Nasogastric tube: It deflates the stomach, reducing the risk of gastric injury during trocar insertion, and improves surgical exposure.
- Urinary catheter to be used for lower abdominal procedures. This decompresses the bladder and reduces the risk of injury.
- Raised intra-abdominal pressure and systemic absorption of carbon dioxide will require increased minute volume and raised airway pressures (maintain normocarbia, $ETCO_2$ near 35 mmHg).
- To watch for inadvertent endobronchial intubation during positioning and creation of pneumoperitoneum.

- Opioids: Short-acting opioids, e.g. fentanyl, alfentanil and remifentanil, can be used intraoperatively to cover what can be an intense but short-lived stimulus.
- Nitrous oxide: Concerns regarding problems with bowel distension and postoperative nausea and vomiting (PONV) have not been substantiated [29].
- Volatiles: Halothane is avoided – sensitizes myocardium in presence of hypercarbia because of risk of arrhythmias. Isoflurane, sevoflurane and desflurane are preferred.
- Gas insufflations into peritoneal cavity with stretching of peritoneum and raised intra-abdominal pressure can cause a range of clinical responses.

Sympathetic responses can be ameliorated by increase in volatile agent concentration, opioids (fentanyl, alfentanil, remifentanil), vasodilators (nitroglycerin drip, IV infusion or spray), beta-blockers (metoprolol) and A2 agonist (dexmedetomidine, clonidine).

- In case of intraoperative hypoxia, the following has to be considered:
  1. Hypoventilation – pneumoperitoneum, position, inadequate ventilation
  2. V/Q mismatch – atelectasis, endobronchial intubation, extraperitoneal gas insufflations, bowel distension, pulmonary aspiration and rarely pneumothorax
  3. Reduced cardiac output – vena caval compression, arrhythmias, haemorrhage, myocardial depression, venous gas embolism and extraperitoneal gas
- Subcutaneous emphysema during procedures spells DANGER – gas insufflations to be checked.
- At the end of operation, the surgeon is encouraged to expel as much CO_2 as possible. To reduce pain, local anaesthesia to be applied to wound sites.
  - Liberal intravenous fluid therapy is preferred to maintain adequate urine output (approximately 10–20 ml/kg/hour), to minimize haemodynamic changes from pneumoperitoneum, to decrease PONV and to improve postoperative recovery [30–32].
  - Choice of intravenous fluid is crystalloid in the form of Ringer-lactate, normal saline and 5% dextrose with normal saline. We usually give 3–4 l of fluid intraoperatively, and average duration of surgery lasts for 3–4 h.

4.4.2.1 Special Consideration for Laparoscopic Donor Nephrectomy

(a) *Urine output*: We overhydrate the donor to maintain urine output >10 ml/kg/hour. We give only crystalloid (NS/RL alternate); if the patient is diabetic, we start dextrose-insulin drip. We try to keep positive fluid balance for around 700 ml to 1 l until the patient is extubated and shifted to the ward.

(b) *Intraoperative haemodynamic*: Due to pneumoperitoneum, it compromises the organ perfusion, including renal, gastrointestinal, liver, etc. To overcome these problems, we try to avoid hypotension and maintain mean arterial blood pressure more than 100 mmHg or maintain vitals 20% more than the baseline.

(c) *Intra-abdominal pressure*: Ideally, intra-abdominal pressure (IAP) needs to be maintained between 12 and 15 mmHg during donor nephrectomy. Sometimes, when it happens due to pneumoperitoneum, renal vessels are in spasm, and urine output is also reduced despite of all effort by the anaesthesiologist; in such a situation, instil papaverine on the renal vessels and keep zero intra-abdominal pressure and wait until you achieve the targeted urine output.

(d) *Diuretics (Frusemide and Mannitol)*: We intermittently give intravenous frusemide (0.75–1 mg/kg) and mannitol (0.25–0.5gm/kg) to maintain urine output. Mannitol is a good osmotic diuretics; it should be given 15–20 min before securing the renal artery. It acts as an osmotic diuretic, preservative and free radical scavenger and minimizes renal vessel spasm by maintaining adequate intravascular osmotic pressure.

(e) *Role of Aminophylline*: It is indicated when donor is a smoker, elderly, compromised or marginal donor kidney (eGFR around 80), we need to overhydrate the patient. It is helpful to prevent renal vessel spasm, mild diuretic action, increase ureteric peristalsis and increase the pulmonary vessels capacitance.

(f) *Heparin*: Some centres use the heparin (3,000–5,000 IU) 10 min before the renal artery clipping [33].

(g) *Sodium bicarbonate*: We give sodium bicarbonate 7.5% 1 ml/kg. It keeps the pH towards the alkali for some time, which is helpful to preserve the donor kidney until perfusion done by cold perfusion fluid.

(h) *Surgical steps*: During CO_2 insufflation, the vitals are monitored, and diuretics given in an incremental dose. Before port placement, injection bupivacaine 0.25% infiltration is necessary to reduce analgesic requirement. Once the surgeon is on the renal hilum dissection, we start mannitol injection in an incremental dose. During adrenal dissection, there is a theoretical possibility of haemodynamic instability in terms of tachycardia which should be kept in mind. We monitor the adequacy of intravascular volume expansion by the turgor of the renal veins. On the recipient side, 20 mg frusemide, 10 mg mannitol and 1 ml/kg sodium bicarbonate are administered for at least 10–15 min prior to retrieval. Meanwhile, the retrieval incision is ready and then surgeons retrieve the kidney. The renal retrieval time, warm ischemia time and cold ischemia time are noted at the conclusion of the procedure. Instillation of 20–40 ml of 0.125–0.25% bupivacaine in the renal fossa will reduce the requirement of postoperative analgesia.

  (i) *Perfusion fluids*: Once the kidney is retrieved, surgeon immediately flushes the kidney with 4–8 °C ice saline and then cold ischemia time will start.

• After the surgery, we extubate the patient on the table. For reversal, we inject a combination of neostigmine (50 mcg/kg) and glycopyrrolate (8 mcg/kg) intravenously. Once all the vitals are stable, we shift the donor to the postoperative ICU.

4.5 Postoperative Management

• In postoperative ICU, patient is monitored for 24 h. All vitals and urine output are noted.
• For intravenous fluid management, equal balance is maintained and crystalloids are preferred.

4.5.1   Postoperative Analgesia

The factors which can be responsible for postoperative pain include port site pain, low abdominal incisions (retrieval incision), pelvic organ nociception, diaphragmatic irritation (shoulder tip discomfort from residual pneumoperitoneum), urinary catheter discomfort, etc.

Pain has a wide spectrum of effects on the body. Incompetently controlled postoperative pain may lead to harmful physiologic and psychological consequences, which increase the morbidity and mortality [34, 35]. It has been recognized that inadequately treated postoperative pain may lead to chronic pain, which is often misdiagnosed and neglected [36, 37].

At our centre, we give on-demand analgesia.

The multimodal analgesic techniques have been shown to control this dynamic pain. For the multimodal approach, we have been following modalities:

(a)   *NSAIDS*:

Nonsteroidal anti-inflammatory drugs (NSAIDs) are generally avoided because of their potential nephrotoxicity and other adverse effects. It was observed that they had the little effect on surgical stress response and organ dysfunction [38, 39]. On the other hand, it was found that NSAIDs provide moderate postoperative analgesia and an opioid-sparing effect in about 20–30% [40]. They can minimize the incidence of opioid-related adverse effects like nausea, vomiting, respiratory depression and ileus and bladder disturbances. If NSAIDs were used for less than 5 days with adequate hydration, they can make a potential alternate to opioids. We do not use NSAIDs in donor nephrectomy patients.

(b)   *Opioid analgesia*:

The use of opioid in postoperative period is a standard practice. At our centre, we use fentanyl, tramadol, pentazocine and nalbuphine. The opioids have associated side effects like postoperative nausea and vomiting (PONV), respiratory depression and sedation. Hence, making use of opioids is far from being the ideal postoperative analgesic of choice following a major surgery like laparoscopic donor nephrectomy.

(c)   *Epidural analgesia*:

Epidural opioids and local anaesthetic (LA) infiltrations have shown that they provide more effective dynamic pain relief. But it is important to note that epidural opioids are less effective on stress response [40].

Continuous epidural administration of local anaesthetic (LA) agents or LA plus opioids was shown to reduce the postoperative pulmonary morbidity after major abdominal surgery [41]. They can also block the sympathetic responses and may reduce the cardiac morbidity [35]. Epidural analgesia was found to be associated with a lower incidence of PONV, sedation and postoperative bowel dysfunction when compared with opioids [42, 43].

(d)   *Transversus abdominis plane (TAP) block*:

This plane is poorly vascularized, and it was found that analgesic effect of TAP block lasts for prolonged duration due to slow drug clearance [44, 45]. But until the date, there is lack of robust data that justifies the efficacy of TAP block for donor laparoscopic nephrectomy.

(e)   *Local long-acting agent infiltration and instillation*:
Pre-emptive port site infiltration can reduce the central sensitization and facilitates recovery by making the earlier ambulation [46–48]. It also reduces the postoperative analgesic requirement. There is lack of properly conducted study in case of donor laparoscopic nephrectomy. Renal fossa instillation with 20 ml 0.5% bupivacaine was found to reduce the requirement of postoperative analgesia in donor laparoscopic nephrectomy.

(f)   *Other modalities* like use of alpha-2 agonist, pregabalin, acetazolamide and antidepressant may minimize the requirement of postoperative analgesia and the side effect related to opioids.

- To prevent postoperative nausea and vomiting, we prefer intravenous injection of 4 mg ondansetron, 10 mg metoclopramide and 40 mg pantoprazole.
- On first postoperative day, we start light diet and early ambulation. On second postoperative day, we start the full diet. Usually, we discharge the donor on third postoperative day.

References

1. Hou S. Expanding the kidney donor pool: ethical and medical consideration. Kidney Int. 2000;58:1820–36.
2. Ellison MD, McBride MA, Taranto SE, et al. Living kidney donors in need of kidney transplants: a report from the organ procurement and transplantation network. Transplantation. 2002;74:1349–51.
3. Davis CL. Evaluation of the living kidney donor: current perspectives. Am J Kidney Dis. 2004;43:503–30.
4. Port FK, Dykstra DM, Merion RM, et al. Trends and results for organ donation and transplantation in united states, 2004. Am J Transplant. 2005;5:843–9.
5. Melcher ML, Carter JT, Posselt A, et al. More than 500 consecutive laparoscopic donor nephrectomies without conversion or repeated surgery. Arch Surg. 2005;140:835–40.
6. Ratner LE, Montgomery RA, Kavoussi LR. Laparoscopic live donor nephrectomy: a review of the first 5 years. Urol Clin North Am. 2001;28:709–19.
7. Lee BR, Chow GK, Ratner LE, et al. Laparoscopic live donor nephrectomy: outcomes equivalent to open surgery. J Endourol. 2000;14:811–9.
8. Jayashree S, Kumra VP. Anaesthesia for laparoscopic surgery. Indian J Surg. 2003;65:232–40.
9. Bardoczky GI, Engelman E, Levarlet M, et al. Ventilatory effects of pneumoperitoneum monitored with continuous spirometry. Anaesthesia. 1993;48:309–11.
10. Fahy BG, Barnas GM, Flowers JL, et al. The effects of increased abdominal pressure on lung and chest wall mechanics during laparoscopic surgery. Anesth Analg. 1995;81:744.
11. Dumont L, Mattys M, Mardirosoff C, et al. Changes in pulmonary mechanics during laparoscopic gastroplasty in morbidly obese patients. Acta Anaesthesiol Scand. 1997;41:408–13.
12. Sprung J, Whalley DG, Falcone T, et al. The impact of morbid obesity, pneumoperitoneum, and posture on respiratory system mechanics and oxygenation during laparoscopy. Anesth Analg. 2002;94:1345.
13. Odeberg-Wernerman S. Laparoscopic surgery – effects on circulatory and respiratory physiology: an overview. Eur J Surg (Suppl). 2000;585:4.
14. Ivankovich AD, Miletich DJ, Albrecht RF, et al. Cardiovascular effects of intraperitoneal insufflation with carbon dioxide insufflation and nitrous oxide in the dog. Anesthesiology. 1975;42:281–7.

15. Takata M, Wise RA, Robotham JL. Effects of abdominal pressure on venous return: abdominal vascular zone conditions. J Appl Physiol. 1990;69:1961–72.

16. Cunningham AJ, Turner J, Rosenbaum S, et al. Transoesophageal echocardiographic assessment of haemodynamic function during laparoscopic cholecystectomy. Br J Anaesth. 1993;70:621–5.

17. Odeberg S, Ljungqvist O, Svenberg T, et al. Haemodynamic effects of pneumoperitoneum and the influence of posture during anaesthesia for laparoscopic surgery. Acta Anaesthesiol Scand. 1994;38:276–83.

18. Giebler RM, Behrends M, Steffens T, et al. Intraperitoneal and retroperitoneal carbon dioxide insufflation evoke different effects on caval vein pressure gradients in humans: evidence for the starling resistor concept of abdominal venous return. Anesthesiology. 2000;92:1568–80.

19. Abassi Z, Bishara B, Karram T, et al. Adverse effects of pneumoperitoneum on renal function: involvement of the endothelin and nitric oxide systems. Am J Physiol Regul Integr Comp Physiol. 2008;294:842–50.

20. Rosenthal RJ, Hiatt JR, Phillips EH, et al. Intracranial pressure: effects of pneumoperitoneum in a large-animal model. Surg Endosc. 1997;11:376–80.

21. Fowkes FJ, Price JF, Fowkes FG. Incidence of diagnosed deep vein thrombosis in general population: systemic review. Eur J Vasc Andovasc Surg. 2003;25:1.

22. Kavoussi LR, Sosa E, Chandhoke P, et al. Complications of laparoscopic pelvic lymph node dissection. J Urol. 1993;149:322.

23. Cadeddu JA, Wolf Jr JS, Nakada S, et al. Complications of laparoscopic procedures after concentrated training in urological laparoscopy. J Urol. 2001;166:2109.

24. Pradoni P, Lensing AW, Cogo A, et al. The long term clinical course of acute deep venous thrombosis. Ann Intern Med. 1996;125:1.

25. Turpie AG, Chin BS, Lip GY. ABC of antithrombotic therapy: venous thromboembolism: pathophysiology, clinical features and prevention. BMJ. 2002;325:887.

26. Neudecker J, Sauerland S, Neugebauer E, et al. The European association for endoscopic surgery clinical practice guideline on the pneumoperitoneum for laparoscopic surgery. Surg Endosc. 2002;16:1121.

27. Gan TJ, Glass PS, Windsor A, et al. Bispectral index monitoring allows faster emergence and improved recovery from propofol, alfentanil and nitrous oxide anesthesia. Anesthesiology. 1997;87:808.

28. Song D, Joshi GP, White PF. Titration of volatile anesthetics using bispectral index facilitates recovery after ambulatory anesthesia. Anesthesiology. 1997;87:842.

29. Knos GB, Sung YF, Toledo A. Pneumopericardium associated with laparoscopy. J Clin Anesth. 1991;3:56–9.

30. Holte K, Klarskov B, Christensen DS, et al. Liberal versus restrictive fluid administration to improve recovery after laparoscopic cholecystectomy: a randomized, double-blind study. Ann Surg. 2004;240:892–9.

31. Magner JJ, McCaul C, Carton E, et al. Effect of intraoperative intravenous crystalloid infusion on postoperative nausea and vomiting after gynaecological laparoscopy: comparison of 30 and 10 ml kg(-1). Br J Anaesth. 2004;93:381.

32. Maharaj CH, Kallam SR, Malik A, et al. Preoperative intravenous fluid therapy decreases postoperative nausea and pain in high risk patients. Anesth Analg. 2005;100:675.

33. Peter J. Morris, Stuart J. Knechtle. Kidney transplantation. 6th ed. Chapter 8B laparoscopic live donor nephrectomy; 2008:119.

34. Joshi GP. Multimodal analgesia techniques and postoperative rehabilitation. Anesthesiol Clin North Am. 2005;23(1):185–202.

35. Liu SS, Carpenter RL, Mackey DC, et al. Effects of perioperative analgesic technique on rate of recovery after colon surgery. Anesthesiology. 1995;83:757–65.

36. Williams M, Milner QJW. Postoperative analgesia following renal transplantation – current practice in the UK. Anaesthesia. 2003;58(7):712–3.

37. Nikolajsen L, Sørensen HC, Jensen TS, et al. Chronic pain following caesarean section. Acta Anaesthesiol Scand. 2004;48(1):111–6.

38. Kehlet H. Multimodal approach to control postoperative pathophysiology and rehabilitation. Br J Anaesth. 1997;78(5):606–17.
39. Kehlet H. Modification of responses to surgery by neural blockade: clinical implications. In: Cousins MJ, Bridenbaugh, editors. Neural blockade in clinical aneathesia and management of pain. 3rd ed. Philadelphia: Lippincott-Raven; 1998. p. 129–71.
40. Kehlet H, Holte K. Effect of postoperative analgesia on surgical outcome. Br J Anaesth. 2001;87(1):62–72.
41. Addison NV, Brear FA, Budd K, et al. Epidural analgesia following cholecystectomy. Br J Surg. 1974;61(10):850–2.
42. Dolin SJ, Cashman JN, Bland JM. Effectiveness of acute postoperative pain management: I. Evidence from published data. Br J Anaesth. 2002;89(3):409–23.
43. Suarez-Sanchez L, Perales-Caldera E, Pelaez-Luna MC, et al. Postoperative outcome of open donor nephrectomy under epidural analgesia: a descriptive analysis. Transplant Proc. 2006;38(3):877–81.
44. McDonnell JG, O'Donnell B, Curley G, Heffernan A, et al. The analgesic efficacy of transversus abdominis plane block after abdominal surgery: a prospective randomized controlled trial. Anesth Analg. 2007;104(1):193–7.
45. McDonnell JG, Curley G, Carneyetal J. The analgesic efficacy of transverses abdominis plane block after caesarean delivery: a randomized controlled trial. Anesth Analg. 2008;106(1):186–91.
46. Vloka JD, Hadzic A, Mulcare R, et al. Femoral and genitofemoral nerve blocks versus spinal anesthesia for outpatients undergoing long saphenous vein stripping surgery. Anesth Analg. 1997;84(4):749–52.
47. Li S, Coloma M, White PF, et al. Comparison of the costs and recovery profiles of three anesthetic techniques for ambulatory anorectal surgery. Anesthesiology. 2000;93(5):1225–30.
48. Song D, Greilich NB, White PF, et al. Recovery profiles and costs of anesthesia for outpatient unilateral inguinal herniorrhaphy. Anesth Analg. 2000;91(4):876–81.

Laparoscopic Left Donor Nephrectomy (Transperitoneal Approach)

Arvind P. Ganpule, Mahesh R. Desai, Gopal Tak, and Abhishek Singh

Abstract

The left side is the preferred renal unit for engrafting. The obvious reasons for this are easier dissection of the hilum, anatomically longer vein. This makes the recipient surgery easier. A longer renal vein offers ease for the recipient surgeon. However, in comparison to the right side, the left side involves a few inherent anatomical challenges, which include the need for dissection of the lumbar vein, the adrenal vein, and the gonadal vein. The left side requires aggressive dissection of the upper pole particularly the spleen. In this chapter, we emphasize on the intricacies in the steps of laparoscopic donor nephrectomy on the left side.

5.1 Introduction

The left side is the preferred renal unit for engrafting. The obvious reasons for this are easier dissection of the hilum, anatomically longer vein. This makes the recipient surgery easier. A longer renal vein offers ease for the recipient surgeon. However, in comparison to the right side, the left side involves a few inherent anatomical challenges, which include the need for dissection of the lumbar vein, the adrenal vein, and the gonadal vein. The left side requires aggressive dissection of the upper pole particularly the spleen. In this chapter, we emphasize on the intricacies in the steps of laparoscopic donor nephrectomy on the left side.

A.P. Ganpule (✉) • M.R. Desai • G. Tak • A. Singh
Muljibhai Patel Urological Hospital, Nadiad, Gujarat, India
e-mail: doctorarvind1@gmail.com

© Springer Nature Singapore Pte Ltd. 2017
M.R. Desai, A.P. Ganpule (eds.), *Laparoscopic Donor Nephrectomy*,
DOI 10.1007/978-981-10-2849-6_5

5.2   The Armamentarium (Figure 5.1-Instruments Trolley)

1. One 10 mm 30° telescope
2. Two 11/12 mm ports (dilating tip trocars)
3. Two 5 mm ports
4. One Maryland forceps
5. Dissecting laparoscopic scissors
6. Single-action or double-action bowel grasper
7. Right-angled laparoscopy forceps
8. Energy sources:
   (a) Ultrasonic Harmonic scalpel™ (optional)
   (b) Bipolar: LigaSure™, ENSEAL™ (optional)
9. Monopolar hook forceps
10. Hemostatic devices
    (a) Hem-o-lok™ clip applicator and clips
    (b) Titanium clip applicator – multiload
    (c) Vascular/Endo GIA stapler – if institutional policy is to use a stapler
11. Open surgical tray and rescue tray

5.3   Procedure- Step by Step

At the outset, the stomach is decompressed with a Ryle's tube, and the bladder emptied with a bladder catheter. Placing the catheter bag at the head end of the patient helps the anesthetist do the monitoring. The patient receives 1–2 liters of

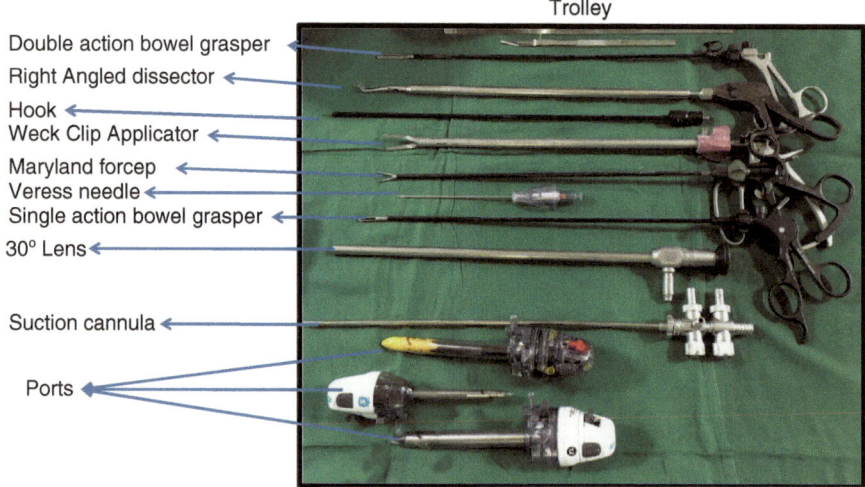

Fig. 5.1 Trolley preparation

intravenous fluid before creating a pneumoperitoneum, and a urine output of 100 cc per hour is ensured throughout the procedure.

CT imaging in form a CT angiography helps in providing a road map for the dissection and completion of the procedure. Apart from providing details regarding the number of vessels (single artery, single vein), it also gives a fair idea regarding the location of the vessels in relation to each other. This information will be gained particularly if the CT images are viewed on the CT console. The same information can be gained if the data is reviewed on a CD. The information offered would be whether the renal artery is caudal or cranial to the renal vein, the number of lumbar veins, and the information regarding the relation of the vein with the artery and lumbar vein.

5.3.1   Patient Positioning (Fig. 5.2)

The patient is placed in right lateral position (left side up). The patient is positioned at the right edge of the table, with the patient's belly hanging down as opposed to the open surgery where the patient is on the left edge of the table for left-sided surgery. Patient is positioned at an angle of $60°$ with the table depending upon the habitus of the patient. The left leg is extended, and right leg flexed with two pillows between the legs; the first pillow is at the level of the thigh placed vertically and other at the level of the leg and the ankle placed horizontally. Patient's back is supported by three cuboid-shaped bolsters. The right arm is extended and kept of an

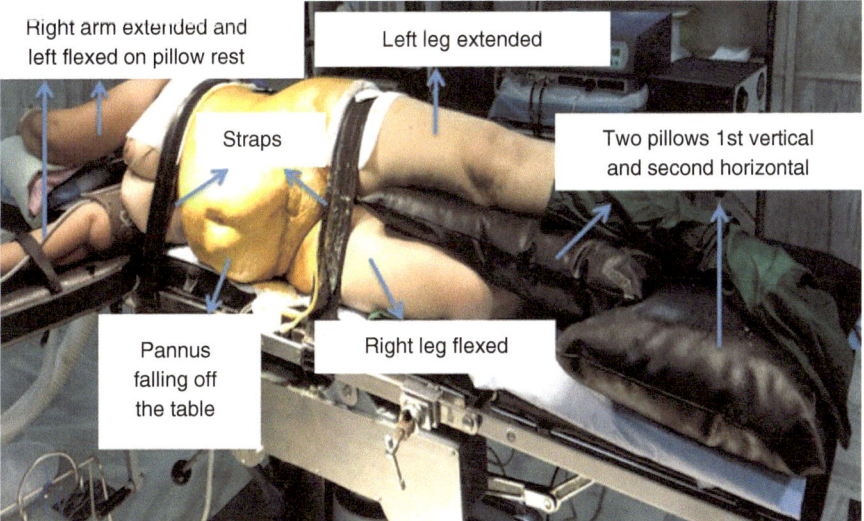

Fig. 5.2 Patient positioning

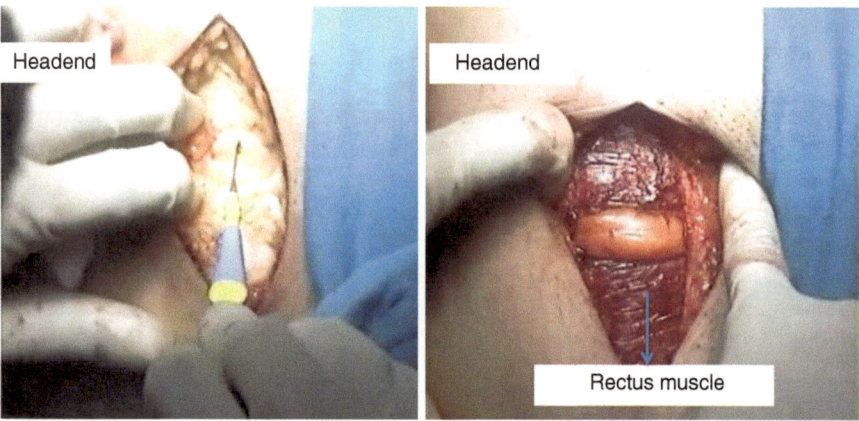

Fig. 5.3 Preplaced extraction incision

arm board after placing an axillary roll; the left arm is flexed at elbow and placed on a mayo's stand or pillow, after placing an axillary roll. Care has to be taken that the patient's left hand is placed in such a way that it does not come in the way of the surgeon's left hand movements, inadvertent pushing of the patient's left hand during surgery may cause a stretch injury to the brachial plexus, and also improper positioning causes limitation of left hand movement of the surgeon. Special attention is paid to securing and strapping pressure points. Padding devices used include commercially available gel pads, cotton rolls, or locally available things like egg crates or foam sheets. The pressure points include the knee, ankle, shoulder, and axilla, and lateral cutaneous nerve of the thigh, the peroneal nerve, and the brachial plexus which are at risk of injury.

The straps are applied on the lower hip and the chest. The straps can be rubber or leather straps available in the market or can be a broad cloth, Elastocrepe, or white cloth sticking. The straps should go all around the patient so that the patient can be rotated during the surgery if required. The anesthetist gives special attention to the strap on the lower chest.

Surgical advantage of such a positioning is that in obese patients the pannus falls away from the operative site and port placement becomes easier.

5.3.2 Preplaced Incision (Fig. 5.3)

A Pfannenstiel incision, which is 5–6 cm in length two to three fingerbreaths above the pubic symphysis pubis, is marked in supine position. A bikini line incision can also be marked in females. The incision is taken once the patient is positioned and prepared. The skin and subcutaneous tissue is incised, and the rectus sheath is opened horizontally and undermined cranially and caudally. Rectus abdominis muscle, pyramidalis muscle, and the midline are identified. The midline is scored with electrocautery, and using an atraumatic forceps and artery forceps, it is split. Preperitoneal fat

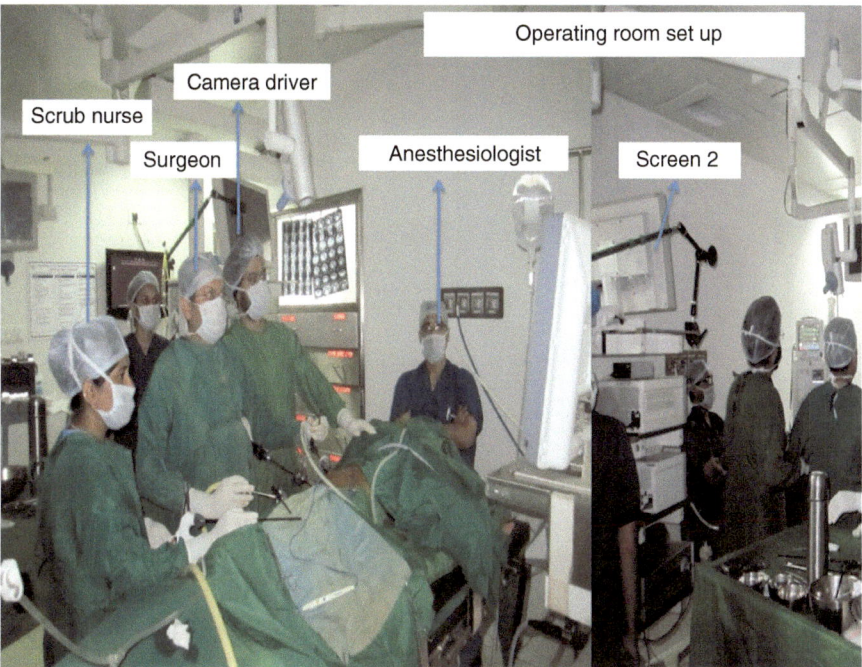

Fig. 5.4 Operating room setup. The figure depicts the position of the surgeon, the assistant, and the anesthetist

is now exposed; using atraumatic forceps and artery forceps, this fat is peeled off from the peritoneum, and peritoneum is thus exposed. The incision is packed with wet mop.

Advantage of this incision is that it can be used in any emergency, vascular accident, where surgeon can use his hand to temporize bleeding. It is a muscle-splitting incision, and hence there are less chances of developing hernia and good healing. Cosmetically, it is a very appealing incision. This incision can be used to train surgeons; the surgeons are allowed to do kidney retrievals from this incision in early part of their training, and when they actually start performing this surgery, they can use this incision in salvaging vascular accidents.

A similar incision can be placed in the left iliac fossa; the disadvantage is that it is a muscle-cutting incision, is less cosmetic, and increases chances of incisional hernia. But it is useful in extremely obese patients and in patients with operative history in lower abdomen.

5.3.3   Operating Room Setup (Fig. 5.4)

The operating surgeon and the camera driver stand on the right of the patient; for most of the situations camera driver standing cranially and surgeon caudally is more ergonomic. The instrument trolley is placed at the foot end of the patient. The scrub

Fig. 5.5 Port positioning

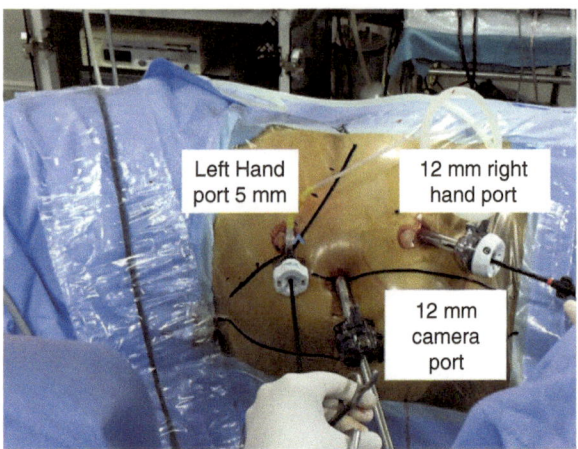

nurse stands caudal to the surgeon. The assistant surgeon stands on the left of the patient and the anesthesiologist at the head end.

The vision cart with the main video monitor is placed in front of the operating surgeon; it should be at a distance, which is equal to five times the diagonal length of monitor. For a 21 inch monitor, the distance of the monitor should be at 105 in. from the surgeon and placed just below the eye level so that the surgeon looks 15° down while operating; this causes the least fatigue on sternocleidomastoid muscle. The insufflator and energy sources should be placed on the vision cart below the monitor so that they are in direct view of the surgeon. The second monitor is placed behind the surgeon so that the assistant can visualize the surgical steps clearly.

5.3.4   Port Placement (Fig. 5.5)

The principles of port positioning include triangulation, positioning the camera in front of the hilum; distance between the two ports is at least four fingerbreaths, so that there is no sword fighting, and the camera port should be midway of the two working ports. The ports should be placed in such a way that the angle between the two working instruments, i.e., the manipulation angle is 60–75°, and the angle between each of the working instrument and the camera, i.e., the azimuth angle, should be between 30 and 45°.

The anterior superior iliac spine (ASIS), the umbilicus, the lateral border of the rectus muscle, midline, subcostal margin, 12th rib, midpoint of the line joining ASIS, and umbilicus are marked using a skin marker. The placement of the port is dictated by the location of the kidney in relation to the costal margin and the truncal obesity.

The first port is indeed at a reference point, which is at the midpoint of the line joining ASIS and the umbilicus. The reference point moves cranially and laterally in obese patients. The first port, which is typically a 12 mm port, is inserted at this reference point. Access technique may vary from institute to institute and patient to patient. In Veress needle technique, the Veress needle is inserted in the abdominal cavity through the point marked for entry of first port. Its position in peritoneal cavity is confirmed by floating ball in the needle hub, change in color indicator to green (both in case of Ethicon™ needles), hanging drop test, and initial pressures of less than 10 mm of Hg. Initial insufflations pressure should be set to 20 mm of Hg, abdomen should be insufflated till it become like tense like a football, and there should be uniform distension and elastic recoil. At this point, one should insert the first port; the direction should be toward the 12th rib keeping it as perpendicular to the abdominal wall as possible. Once the port is inserted, the camera is inserted, and a check peritoneoscopy is done to rule out any injury. The second 5 mm port is placed under vision, below the costal margin in the same line as the first port. The distance between the first two ports should be at least 15 cm; if less, then the second port should be moved medially and cranially till a point that this distance becomes 15 cm. The third or the camera port is again a 12 mm port placed at lateral border of rectus muscle, it is placed at a point which is the junction of cranial one third and caudal two third of the line joining first and the second port. This is exactly in front of the hilum. The vantage location is absolutely essential as this helps in unhindered dissection of the hilum. Some centers use an initial 5 mm port, inspect the peritoneal cavity with 5 mm laparoscope, put the other ports under vision, and then replace the first port with a 12 mm port. The idea of doing this is that if the first port causes an injury, it should be of a lesser magnitude. The fourth port is a 5 mm retraction port placed later in the course of the surgery; it is placed one or two fingerbreath above the ASIS and is used to retract uretero-gonadal packet, lower pole of kidney, and sometimes the upper pole.

In patients who have had multiple previous surgeries, Hasson's technique of port placement under direct vision can be used.

5.3.5   The Bowel Reflection (Figs. 5.6a and b)

On peritoneoscopy, one may find adhesions, which can be in the form of omentum or colon itself stuck to the anterior abdominal wall covering the spleen. These adhesions need to be taken down so that all the landmarks, namely, the spleen, colon, and white line of Toldt, become visible. To incise these adhesions, omental or colonic fat should be held on a stretch and cut close to the abdominal wall using cold scissors. Incising the white line of Toldt remains the first but the most important step of this procedure. The incision along the white line of Toldt is started at the level of kidney, extended toward the spleen and diaphragm cranially and up to the pelvic brim caudally. The key point remains to maintain the plane of dissection in the extra-Gerotal plane. The avascular plane between the Gerota's fascia and the colonic mesentery is developed and followed. The bright globular fat of colonic mesentery is separated from glistening, shining, smooth yellow look of Gerota's fascia with fat within it.

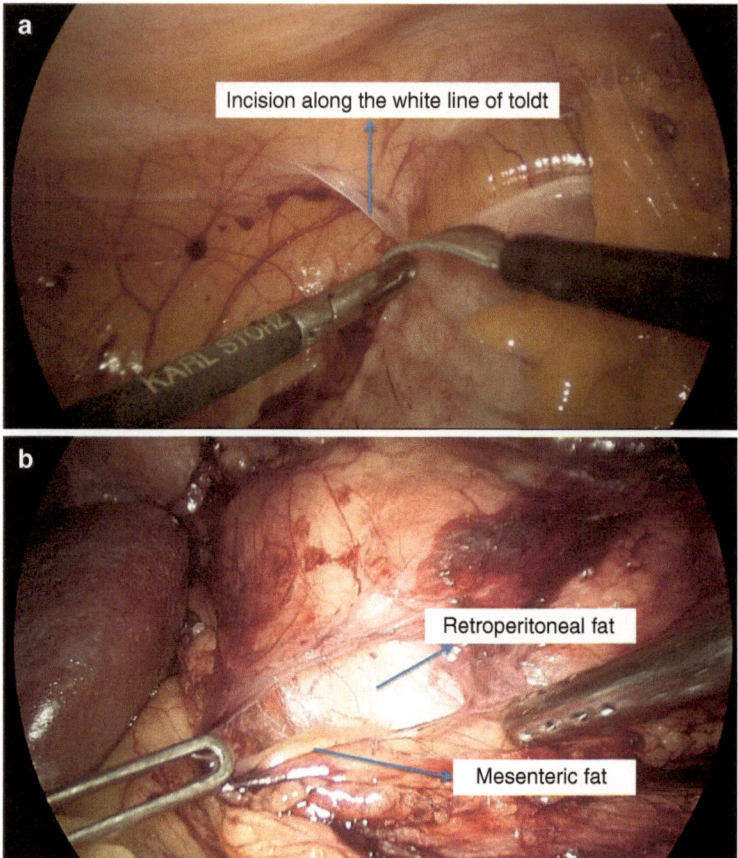

Fig. 5.6 (**a**) Bowel reflection (**b**) Figure showing difference between retroperitoneal and mesenteric fat

The instruments used during this step of surgery include a combination of blunt and sharp instruments. Typically this job can be done with a scissors and suction. The plane should be found till the splenorenal ligament. The newer bipolar devices such as Harmonic scalpel™/LigaSure™ help in dissection in this part of the operation. During reflection of the colon, it is prudent to avoid use of energy close to the colon.

Mesentery is bluntly dissected medially; any bleeding indicates a wrong plane either violation of mesentery or Gerota's fascia. The dissection should be carried cranially where one may encounter more than one plane. Here, using a closed bowel grasping forceps, one should retract the spleen and cut the lienorenal ligament using an energy source like Harmonic scalpel™. This should be done right up to the diaphragm, and in the cranial part of dissection, one should be careful not to injure the stomach or the diaphragm.

Once this is done, the spleen and splenic flexure fall away. This is followed by separation of spleen and pancreas on one side and the upper pole on other.

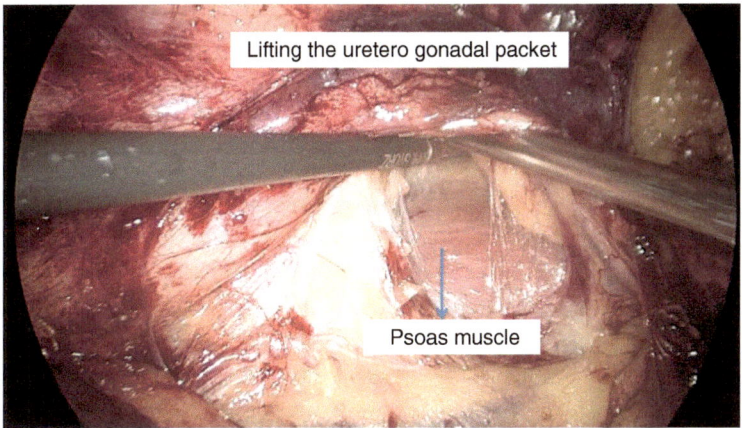

Fig. 5.7 Uretero-gonadal packet

5.3.6   Uretero: Gonadal Packet (Fig. 5.7)

As the mesentery is reflected medially, one may be able to identify the gonadal vein. In case of difficulty, one should try to trace the gonadal vein from the pelvic brim where it is better visible. Once the gonadal vein is seen, the dissection is extended between gonadal vein and colonic mesentery. The mnemonic "water flows below the bridge" helps in identification of the ureter. Ureter is identified by its course, peristalsis, and the vascular pattern around it. The key remains to avoid skeletonizing the ureter. The uretero-gonadal packet should be lifted en bloc. The dissection should not proceed in between the ureter and the gonadal vein. Once the plane is found in between the psoas muscle and the uretero-gonadal packet, the ureter is lifted off the psoas muscle leaving the glistening psoas fascia on the psoas muscle. The dissection then proceeds toward the upper pole remaining on the aorta. An additional port is inserted in the left iliac fossa. The port is 5 mm and helps in introduction of a retracting instrument.

5.3.7   Separation of the Fibrofatty Tissue up to the Renal Hilum

The dissection proceeds on the aorta (identified by the pulsations). Typically, a small twig of the ureteral blood supply will be encountered during this step, which preferentially can be taken with a clip (interlocking metal clip or a polymer 5 mm Hem-o-lok™ clip). The renal vein will be identified by its bluish hue. The preoperative CT helps in identification of the renal vein. The relative location of the entry of the gonadal vein into the renal vein helps in identifying the takeoff of the adrenal vein from the renal vein.

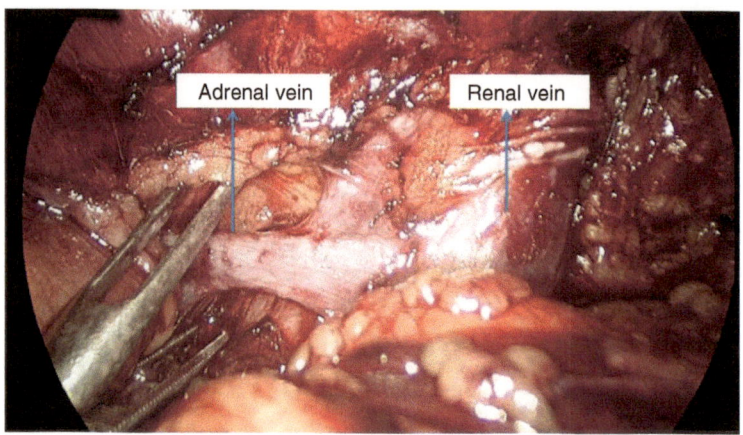

Fig. 5.8 Exposing the Adrenal Vein and Renal vein

5.3.8   Exposing the Renal and the Adrenal Vein (Fig. 5.8)

Once the Gerota's fascia is cleared of the anterior surface of the renal vein, the adrenal vein is identified. The dissection of the adrenal vein should proceed to the point that the adrenal gland is seen. The attempt should be to maintain a significant amount of adrenal vein on the renal vein side. In addition, special care should be taken of the inferior phrenic vein which arises from the adrenal vein. The adrenal vein should be circumferentially dissected and clipped. The clips of choice for clipping adrenal vein are the interlocking clips (metallic) and the polymer clips.

5.3.9   Adrenal Gland Dissection

Once the adrenal vein is secured, a plane is developed between the adrenal gland and the kidney by following the edge of adrenal gland. It is a key point to remain near the adrenal gland and not the kidney; this part of the dissection is intra-Gerotal. The landmarks to be followed include the psoas muscle, kidney, and the adrenal gland. Once the adrenal gland is dissected of the kidney, the upper pole of the kidney is clearly visible, the posterior layer of the Gerota's fascia is now opened by blunt and sharp dissection, and the abdominal wall gets exposed. At this point, the upper pole becomes free and can be lifted up. This part of the dissection proceeds with the help of energy devices such as Harmonic™ or LigaSure™. The advantage of using these energy devices is that they secure small vessels from the splenorenal ligament.

5.3.10 Lumbar Vein Dissection (Fig. 5.9)

The dissection of the lumbar vein is done after the dissection of the upper pole because an inadvertent injury to these veins at a stage wherein the upper pole is

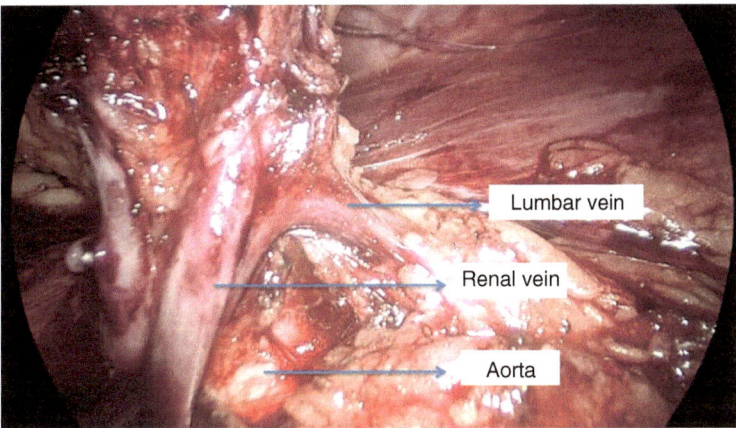

Fig. 5.9 The lumbar vein dissection

not dissected may lead to a potential need to convert to open approach. To dissect the lumbar vein, one needs to identify the lower border of the renal vein. To do this, the assistant lifts the lower pole of the kidney; with an oblique lens, the tissue posterior to the renal vein is visualized. At this point, the aorta and the renal vein ostium are identified. Lumbar vein is identified and dissected for some length toward psoas muscle; many times lumbar vein is broad and has more than one branch. All the branches should be dissected away from the underlying renal artery and then clipped using titanium clips. The lumbar vein is secured away from the renal vein. Adequate cuff of tissue should be kept beyond the clip on the graft side. All attempts should be made to secure the lymphatic tissue in this region.

Once lumbar vein is tackled, the renal artery gets exposed. The artery should be dissected along its length to identify its course and caliber at this stage.

5.3.11 Dissecting the Upper Border of Renal Vein (Fig. 5.10)

The tough tissue cranial to the upper border of the vein is a neuronal tissue. This tissue should be secured once the ostium of the renal artery is clearly seen. The additional port inserted from the iliac fossa help in delineating the vessels.

5.3.12 Renal Arterial Dissection (Fig. 5.11)

The periarterial, lymphatic, and fibrofatty tissue is gradually cut using a hook or Harmonic scalpel; this skeletonizes the renal artery up to its origin from the aorta. Circumferential dissection is completed using a right-angled dissector. Dissection should not be extended to the renal sinus. Minor bleed may occur at this stage, which can be managed by compression, Surgicel™, and occasional use of clips.

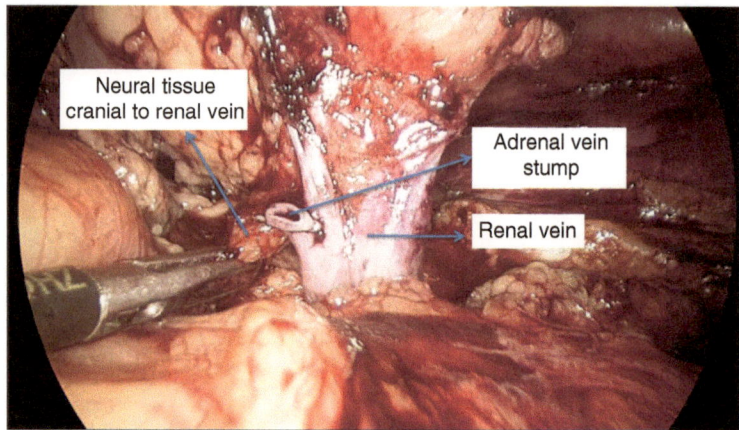

Fig. 5.10 The upper border of renal vein dissection

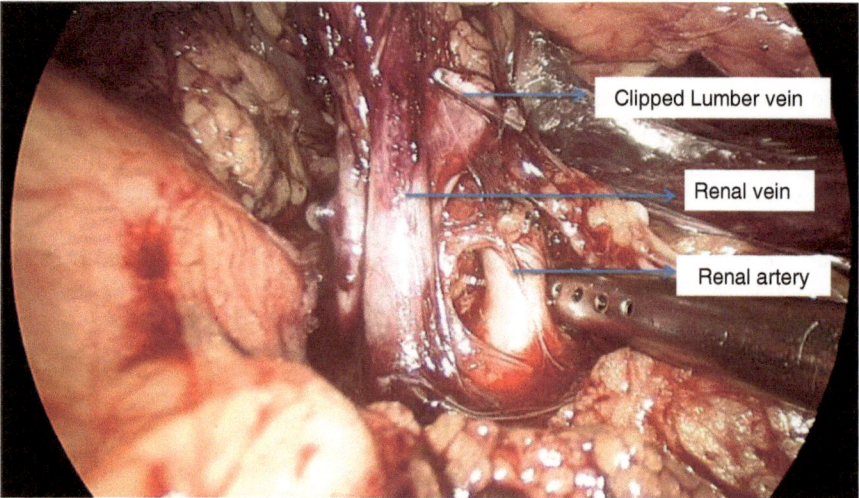

Fig. 5.11 Renal arterial dissection

5.3.13 Renal Vein Dissection (Fig. 5.11)

Renal vein by this time is dissected all around one just needs to pass a right-angled dissector around the renal vein to ensure circumferential dissection.

5.3.14 Retrieval Incision

The issues related to retrieval are discussed elsewhere in the text. The options available include Pfannenstiel, Gibson, or extension of the port.

5.3.15 The Retrieval (Fig. 5.12)

Many surgeons routinely do instillation of papaverine on renal artery; most of the surgeons do not do a systemic heparinization prior to clipping of renal artery. The retrieval starts with securing the gonadal vein; it is secured with the help of interlocking clips. Adequate prudence should be exercised to avoid skeletonization of the ureter while securing this vessel. All attempts should be made to keep adequate amount of tissue with the ureter. Once the gonadal is secured, the ureter should be secured at the level of the iliac crossing. Typically a ureteric artery is encountered at this point. This should be looked for and secured. The ureter is secured with clips. On transection of the ureter, an adequately perfused graft shows a spurt of urine.

The next step is to detach the kidney from the posterior surface. This step should be left for the last, as an earlier detachment of the posterior attachment of the kidney will make the dissection of the hilum challenging. The proper plane for this dissection should be identified. This is typically extra-Gerotal. A consistent muscular feeder is seen arising from the posterior abdominal wall entering the Gerota's fascia; it should be cauterized. The superior portion of the kidney should be separated from the posterior abdominal wall. At this stage the kidney hangs from a small lateral attachment, which is disconnected at last.

Thereafter, the renal hilum is secured. The ostium of the artery should be secured at the level of the aorta by using two Hem-o-lok™ clips, which are placed at a distance on 1–2 mm from each other. The artery is cut leaving a margin of 1–2 mm beyond the clip. Similarly, the renal vein should be secured below the adrenal vein using two Hem-o-lok™ clip placed at a distance of 1–2 mm from each other. Renal

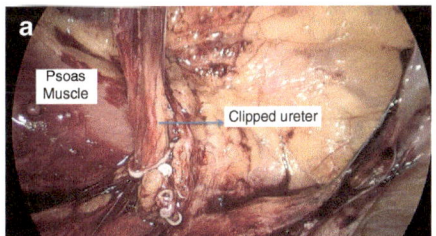
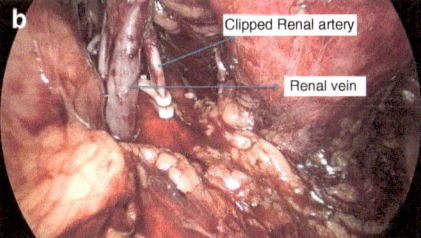
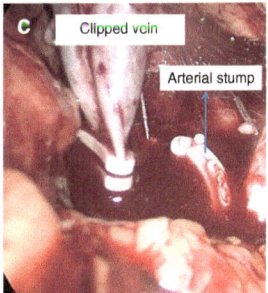

Fig. 5.12 (a–c) Retrieval

vein is cut after leaving a cuff of 1–2 mm beyond the clip. The application of the first arterial clip marks the beginning of warm ischemia. The key to safe retrieval is adequate exposure. The fourth port forms the assistant aids in this. Any remnant tissue posterior to the artery is secured with Hem-o-lok™ clips. The kidney is separated away from residual attachments. Once the kidney is freed, it is held by a grasper, and the assistants expose the wound using c-shaped retractors. The retrieval surgeon is wearing a nonporous arm guard up to the elbow; he incises the peritoneum, enters the peritoneum, and under vision catches the lower pole of the kidney; the grasper holding the kidney is released and retrieval completed. Kidney is placed in ice slush, and this marks the beginning of the cold ischemia, while retrieval care should be taken not to injure the kidney with the edges of the port.

The retrieval surgeon places a mop in the renal fossa and looks for hemostasis. If there is no active bleeding, wound is closed up to the level of rectus sheath, and a check laparoscopy performed.

5.3.16 Hem-o-lok Clip

These are polymer clips available in three sizes: 5 mm (green), 10 mm (purple), and 15 mm (gold). There has been a black box warning regarding the use of these clips in laparoscopic donor nephrectomy. This was issued following reports of deaths from improper use of these clips in donor nephrectomy.

5.3.17 Check Laparoscopy

Pneumoperitoneum is recreated and renal hilum inspected for bleeding. Other potential areas of bleeding like the adrenal bed, ureteric stump, gonadal vein, and abdominal wall are inspected. Abdominal cavity is irrigated with normal saline, which is completely sucked out. Wound is inspected from within, and pelvic collections are sucked out. Ports are closed using Carter-Thomason needle with Vicryl™ no. 1 suture, ports are inspected for bleeding, and finally skin is closed with Monocryl™ 3-0.

Laparoscopic Right Donor Nephrectomy (Transperitoneal Approach)

6

Nariman Ahmadi and Monish Aron

Abstract

Laparoscopic donor nephrectomy has gained significant momentum in recent years with the aim of minimizing postoperative morbidity as well as enhancing the recovery of the donors. Laparoscopic right donor nephrectomy continues to be performed less often despite increased uptake of laparoscopy in recent years. This has been due to combination of factors, which includes short length of the right renal vein, technical challenge and the poor graft survival in the early years.

In this chapter we briefly examine the issues regarding laparoscopic right donor nephrectomies and describe a step-by-step approach in performing laparoscopic transperitoneal right donor nephrectomy.

6.1 Introduction

Laparoscopic donor nephrectomy is a zero-error operation for which the safety of the donor has to be considered above all. Donors who undergo open donor nephrectomy forgo significant portion of their annual income, experience significant pain, and pay out-of-pocket expenses for travel, housing, and childcare. Prolonged recuperative time, pain, and cosmetic results are, therefore, disincentives to traditional live kidney donation. Feasibility of laparoscopic donor nephrectomy was initially reported in 1995 by Ratner and colleagues with the aim of

N. Ahmadi • M. Aron (✉)
University of Southern California, Los Angeles, CA, USA
e-mail: monisharon@hotmail.com

© Springer Nature Singapore Pte Ltd. 2017
M.R. Desai, A.P. Ganpule (eds.), *Laparoscopic Donor Nephrectomy*,
DOI 10.1007/978-981-10-2849-6_6

minimizing morbidity as well as improving recovery parameters [1]. Since then, laparoscopic donor nephrectomy has become an established alternative to the traditional open approach [2]. Whether open or laparoscopic, the left kidney is often favored to the right. This is mainly attributed to the short right renal vein and early experiences of renal vein thrombosis and graft loss [2]. Consequently right donor nephrectomy is performed in only 5–15 % of all laparoscopic donor nephrectomy series [3–5]. Several indications do prompt consideration of the right over the left kidney for donation, and the incorporation of right kidney donation will maximize the transplant pool. However, laparoscopic right donor nephrectomy has been the cause of trepidation even in the hands of the most experienced minimally invasive surgeons.

Recent and more contemporary series have demonstrated the safety and feasibility of this procedure for the donor as well as equivalent graft survival and function for the recipient [3]. A recent meta-analysis by Wang et al. revealed no differences in graft function or loss, conversion to open nephrectomy, and donor or recipient postoperative complication rates [6]. More interestingly, the right donor nephrectomy group had shorter operative time, intraoperative complications, and blood loss. At our institution we advocate performing laparoscopic right donor nephrectomy, if clinically appropriate. This procedure should be performed by experienced laparoscopic surgeons who in turn should be familiar with open donor nephrectomy, should the need arise. In this chapter we describe our technique of donor nephrectomy in a stepwise manner and pay particular attention to points of techniques in each step.

6.2 Step-by-Step Approach

6.2.1 Preoperative Preparation and Evaluation

Prior to this procedure, all patients should undergo the comprehensive donor workup, which has been discussed in the previous chapters. Surgeons need to familiarize themselves with the vascular anatomy on the CT angiography prior to start of the procedure. The CT scans should be displayed in the operating room throughout the procedure. The site of the surgery should be marked, the consent form reviewed, and patient's questions addressed prior to the start of the case. Patients should be well hydrated with satisfactory urine output. Needless to say, it is the responsibility of the surgeon to perform the final check to ensure all safety parameters are addressed prior to initiation of the procedure. Furthermore, the open nephrectomy surgical tray should be available in the operating room during the procedure, and nursing staff should be well trained and familiar with emergent conversion protocols should the need arise. Major bleeding from the right renal vein and IVC are catastrophic events, and all precautions should be taken to be well prepared should this happen.

6.2.2   Positioning Patient and Room Setup

Operating room setup has been shown in Fig. 6.1. The surgeon and the assistant stay on the left side of the patient and the scrub nurse as well as the tower on the right side. The surgeon and the assistant positions may vary depending on the comfort and preference; however, we recommend the surgeon standing caudally to the assistant for ergonomic reasons. The main video monitor should be directly in front of surgeon and at eye level. Surgeon should also have view of the laparoscopic tower including the diathermy settings and the insufflator pressure monitors. Additional monitors should be available for the anesthetist as well as the scrub nurse.

Patients should have an indwelling catheter (IDC) and DVT prophylaxis measures such as pneumatic calf compression device and subcutaneous heparin. Prior to positioning, the site for the Pfannenstiel incision (2–3 cm above pubic symphysis, 5–6 cm length) is marked as this will change once the patient is placed in flank position. This is particularly important in more obese donors. The IDC bag should be placed at the head end of the bed for urine output monitoring by the anesthetist during the case.

Patients are positioned in a 45–60-degree left lateral position with the right side up; a 1 L saline bag is positioned under the axilla to avoid brachial plexus

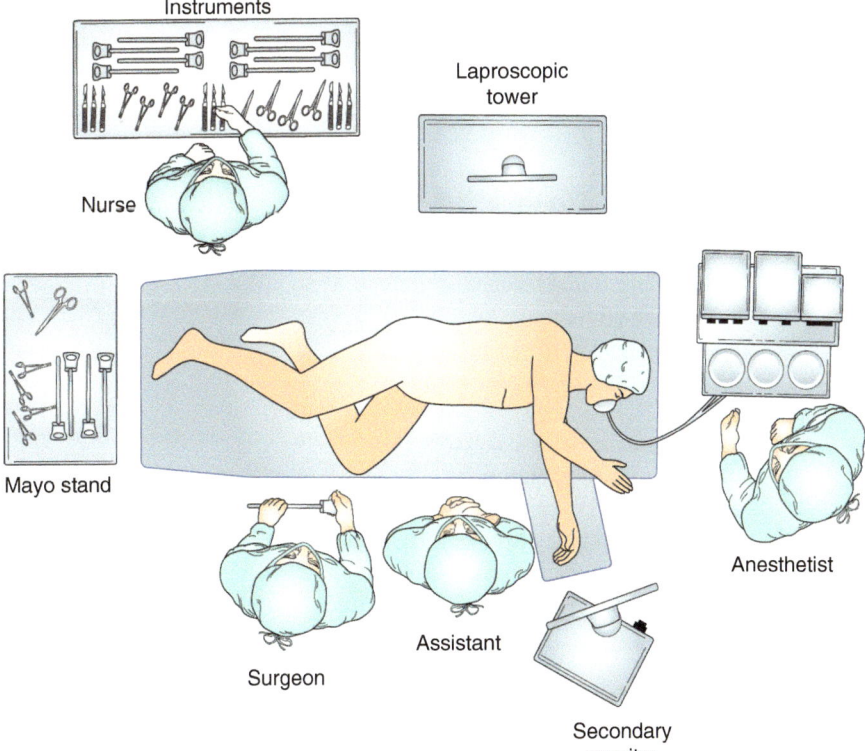

Fig. 6.1 Showing patient positioning

neuropraxia. We do not use the kidney rest routinely. The patient is placed at the edge of the bed and secured with tapes to the bed at the level of iliac crest and mid-thorax. We utilize the 3 in. Leukoplast (BSN medical) as it provides firm grip and does not stretch. Surgeons should ensure that the patient is secure, in case bed rotation is required during the case. Care is taken to protect the nipples as well as the penis from the adhesive tapes. Once the patient is secured to the bed, the arms are placed in their final position. The left arm is extended and rested on an armrest in neutral position, and the right arm is flexed and positioned on an armrest with elbows at same level with angle of the mandible. This positioning of the right arm allows the surgeon's right arm not to clash with the patient's right elbow during the procedure which in turn allows for improved access during dissection of the lower pole and the distal ureter. Skin preparation should be extended to include the site for the Pfannenstiel incision as well as the flank should the need for conversion to open surgery arise. We place the camera cord, light source, as well as the insufflation tube cranially and all other tubes and cords caudally. We place two long quivers on the lateral edge of the drape for secure placements of laparoscopic instruments during the case.

6.2.3   The Armamentarium (Fig. 6.2)

1. Ports:
   (a) 2 × 5 mm ports
   (b) 3 × 12 mm port
   (c) 1 × 15 mm port
2. 10 mm 30-degree telescope
3. Graspers:
   (a) 1× small bowel grasper
   (b) 1× bullet nose forceps
   (c) 1× short fenestrated forceps
   (d) 1× right-angled forceps
   (e) 1× laparoscopic Satinsky clamp
   (f) 1× laparoscopic 10 mm fan retractor
4. Energy devices
   (a) Dissecting laparoscopic scissors
   (b) Monopolar hook diathermy
5. Hemostasis devices:
   (a) Hem-o-lok® (Teleflex Medical, NC, USA) applicator and clips
   (b) Titanium clip applicator and clips
   (c) Vascular endoscopic stapling device (Endo TA 30 mm)
6. Open surgical tray

6.2.4   Port Placements (Fig. 6.3)

The main objective of port placements is optimum vision of the renal hilum. The camera port is a 12 mm port positioned at the lateral edge of the rectus

Trolley

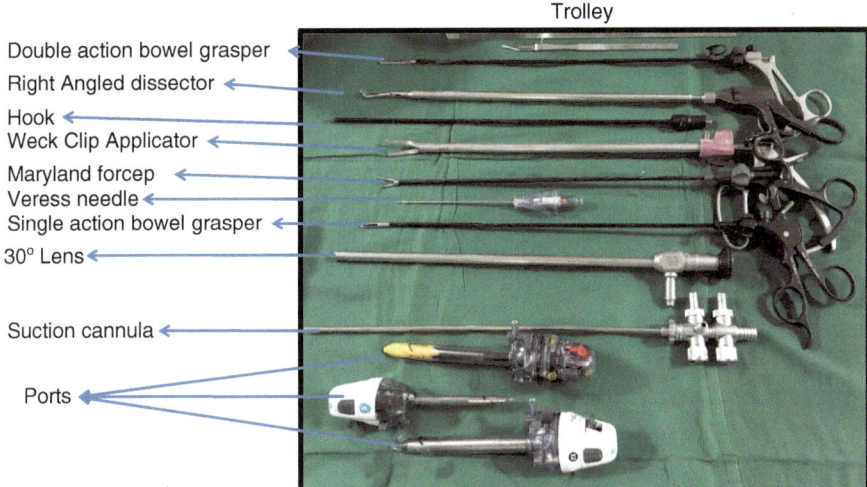

Double action bowel grasper

Right Angled dissector

Hook
Weck Clip Applicator

Maryland forcep
Veress needle
Single action bowel grasper

30° Lens

Suction cannula

Ports

Fig. 6.2 Showing laparoscopic instrumentation required

Fig. 6.3 Showing port positioning

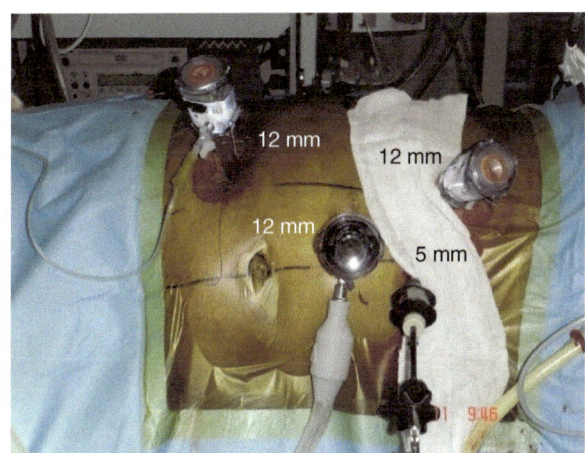

12 mm

12 mm

12 mm

5 mm

muscle, 2 cm caudal to the transpyloric plane. This should translate intra-abdominally to just below the level of the renal hilum. Surgeons must always correlate this port position with the CT scan and individualize the position accordingly. We utilize the Veress needle technique which has been described in the previous chapter. The next stage is performing a diagnostic laparoscopy and inspection of the abdomen for any injury related to the entry technique as well as the presence of any abdominal pathology. The camera port is the reference port, and the remaining ports position may vary depending on the patient's body habitus. All ports should be at least 4–5 cm away from each other to avoid instrument clashing. The lower working port (12 mm) is placed between the umbilicus and iliac crest about 2 cm lateral to the midaxillary line. The slight lateral positioning of this port facilitates better retraction of the kidney as well as posterior dissection of the renal hilum. The upper working port (5 mm) is placed along the midaxillary line about 2 cm below the costal margin. A third 5 mm port is placed 4 cm below the xiphisternum and is used to aid in superior retraction of the liver. Occasionally, an additional 5 mm port could be placed which will aid in renal retraction and exposure of the renal hilum so that the surgeon may utilize both arms in performing the dissection. In our experience, the position of this port is optimal at 4 cm lateral to midpoint of the working ports (Image 2). Prior to start of the case, the height of the bed is adjusted to ensure the surgeon's shoulders are relaxed. This will aid in prevention of fatigue and optimal surgical ergonomics.

6.2.5   **Exposure** (Figs. 6.4 and 6.5)

The first step of the dissection is to provide adequate exposure. Through the xiphisternal port, a ratcheted grasper is deployed underneath the right and left liver lobes as well as the gallbladder to grasp the lateral diaphragmatic muscles for cephalad retraction of the liver for better access and visualization for the upper pole of the kidney. During this step utmost care should be taken to avoid injury of the liver, perforations of the gallbladder, as well as grasping of the intercostal nerves. Occasionally adhesions of the omentum to the gallbladder could be encountered. These adhesions should be divided for optimal view; once again surgeons should be careful of injury to the gallbladder including thermal injury through heat conduction. The right triangular ligaments of the liver should also be divided to allow a better cephalad retraction and slight clockwise rotation of the right liver. Other omental adhesions to the abdominal wall should also be dissected prior to mobilization of the right colon. It is not unusual to encounter adhesions in right lower quadrant, most commonly due to previous appendectomy.

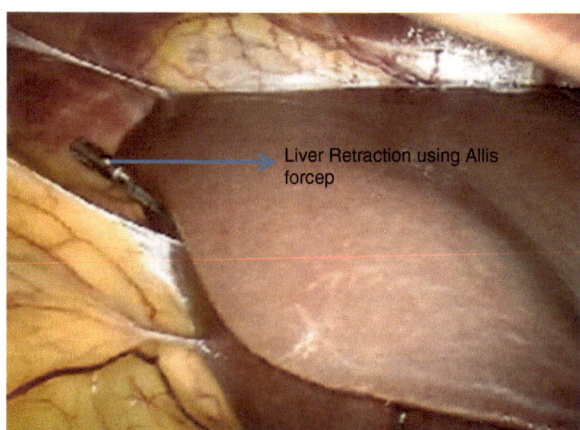

Fig. 6.4 Shows the laparoscopic view of the liver being retracted by Allis forceps

6.2.6   Medialization of the Colon and Duodenum (Figs. 6.6 and 6.7)

The right colon is medialized by incising the lateral peritoneal reflection of Toldt. Keeping the lateral attachments of the kidney intact is a key step which results in suspension of the kidney. This in turn aids in hilar dissection at later stage. It is

Fig. 6.5 Laparoscopic view on the right side

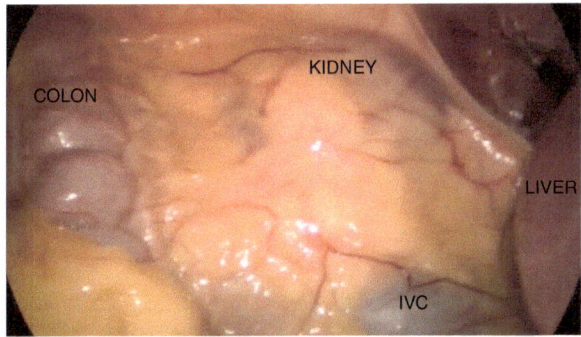

Fig. 6.6 Showing distinction between colonic fat and retroperitoneal fat

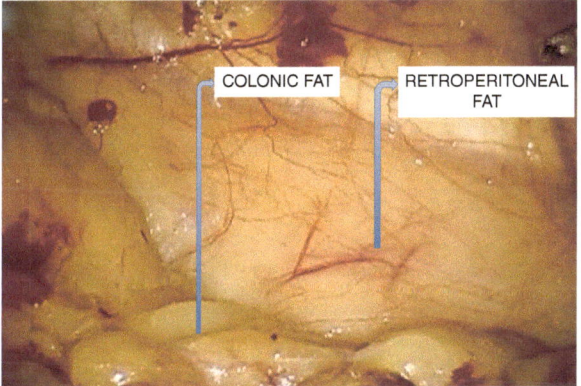

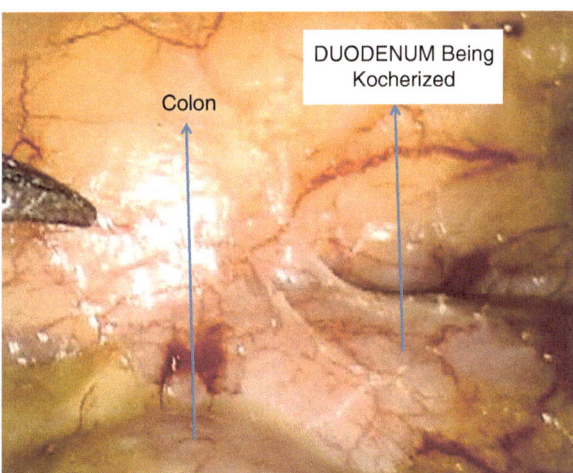

Fig. 6.7 Showing colonic mobilization and duodenal Kocherization

paramount to identify the avascular plane between the colonic mesentery and the Gerota's fascia. The two could be distinguished from one another by the color and contour of the fat. Colon mobilization should extend to the level of the iliac vessels so that the colon passively reflects downward and out of the way from the renal hilar field. Surgeons should now take a moment to identify and distinguish the IVC from the duodenum. The duodenum is now Kocherized in order to expose the IVC as well as the renal hilum. In this step, it is best to lift the fibers just lateral to the edge of the duodenum up and away from IVC and preferably perform sharp dissection. Thermal dissection is minimized, and the surgeons should avoid excessive manipulation and handling of the duodenum. Furthermore, duodenum should always be dissected prior to dissection of the IVC.

6.2.7 Dissection of the IVC

Prior to dissection of the IVC, surgeons should inspect and identify the approximate position of the right renal vein as well as the right gonadal vein (Fig. 6.8a, b). It is of note that the origin of the right gonadal vein is usually on the anterior (rather than lateral) aspect of the IVC, about 1–2 cm below the renal vein. The IVC is now dissected along its anterior and lateral aspect to fully expose the origin of the right renal vein and the right gonadal vein. Meticulous care and dissection techniques are mandatory to avoid thermal injury and bleeding from the IVC. We do not routinely divide the gonadal vein; however, if injured it could be ligated and divided with impunity.

6.2.8 Dissection of the Ureter (Fig. 6.9a, b)

The dissection is now carried out just lateral to the right gonadal vein and the lateral edge of IVC (Fig. 6.10) and extended caudally. The ureter and the periureteric tissue are retracted laterally, and blunt dissection is performed until the psoas sheath is

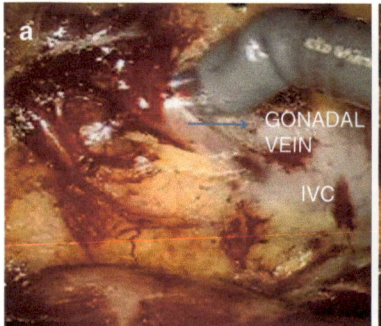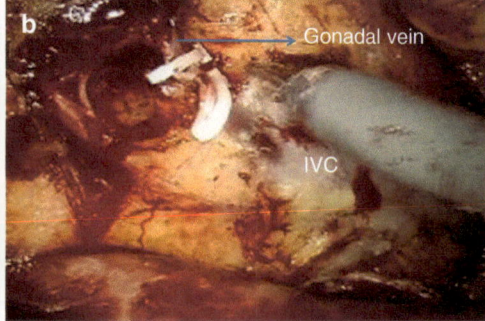

Fig. 6.8 (a, b) Showing the gonadal vein being dissected and clipped

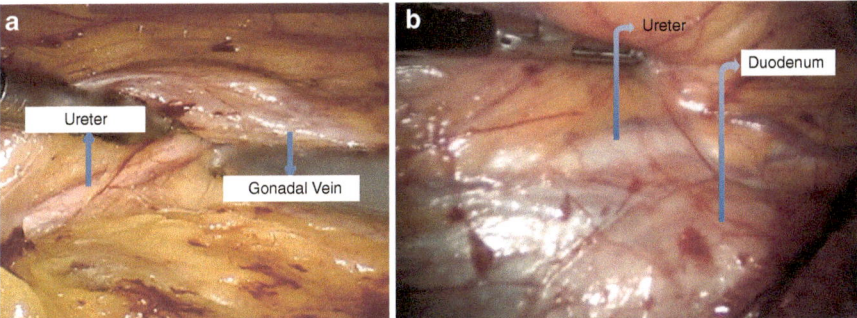

Fig. 6.9 (**a**, **b**) Showing the ureter and lifted ureterogonadal packet

Fig. 6.10 Showing
exposed psoas muscle and
IVC after ureterogonadal
packet is lifted

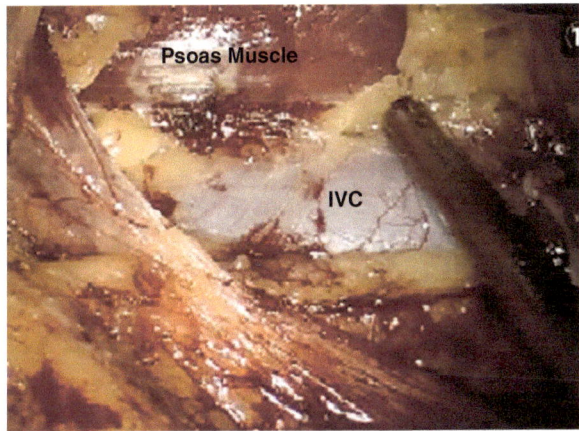

identified. The ureter and its periureteric fat are all reflected upward and away from
the psoas muscle by placing a grasper underneath. From the lateral 5 mm port, the
space created between posterior Gerota's fascia and psoas sheath extended caudally
and cranially from the pelvic brim to the posterior kidney. Manual handling of the
ureter and thermal dissection at close vicinity to the ureter must be avoided at all
times. Preservation of the periureteric tissue is paramount in preserving the distal
ureteric blood supply.

6.2.9   Dissection of the Adrenal Gland (Fig. 6.11a, b)

The dissection is now carried out superior to the renal hilum (Fig. 6.11a). The peritoneal attachments between the kidney and the edge of the liver are divided in order
to provide further cephalad retraction of the liver. This will further expose the upper
pole of the kidney as well as the adrenal. The Gerota's fascia is incised along the
interface between the adrenal gland and the kidney. In this step, a hemostatic dissection is necessary as there are many small veins communicating from renal tissue to

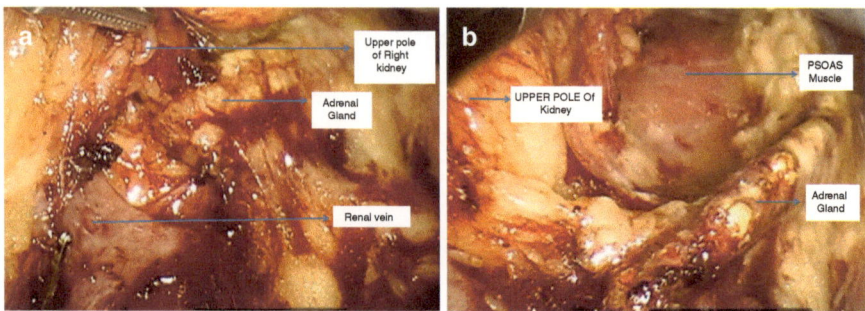

Fig. 6.11 (**a, b**) Showing renal vein identification, upper pole dissection, exposure of the psoas muscle, and upper pole being dissected away from the adrenal gland

Fig. 6.12 The renal artery and renal vein completely dissected

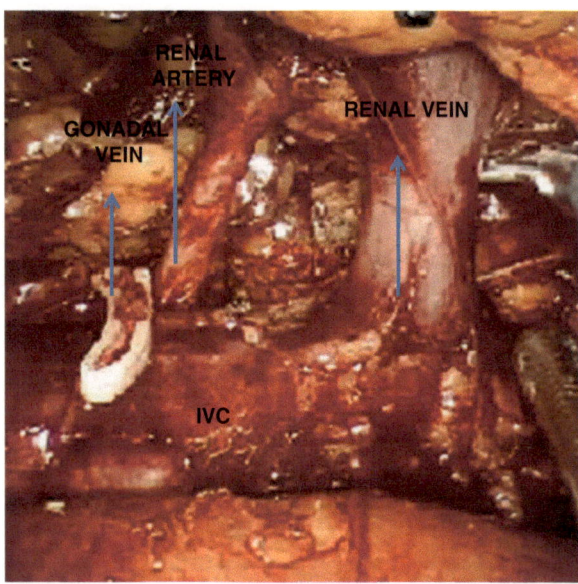

the adrenal gland. Dissection should be carried close to the adrenal gland rather than the kidney and extended laterally to the abdominal wall (Fig. 6.11b). The posterior spaces created between psoas sheath and Gerota's fascia, cranial and caudal to the renal hilum, should communicate at this stage, and the only remaining attachments should be the renal hilum and the lateral attachments.

6.2.10 Dissection of Hilar Vessels (Fig. 6.12)

Prior to hilar dissection, the surgeon should once again confirm the vascular anatomy from the preoperative CT scan. The renal artery can be divided either at the retrocaval space or alternatively at the interaortocaval space. The latter is the preferred option for cases in which there is retrocaval branching of the renal artery; otherwise, a retrocaval approach should yield a satisfactory length of the renal artery for transplantation. Further lateral and posterior dissection of IVC is needed in order to expose the retrocaval portion of the right renal artery. Small fibrofatty and lymphatic tissues around the artery are dissected carefully. Care should be taken to avoid dissection of the renal artery close to the renal sinus as this may result in vasospasm and graft dysfunction. Also the surgeon needs to be wary of excessive traction as well as inadvertent thermal injury to the vessels. If the renal artery is to be divided at the interaortocaval space, the duodenum should be Kocherized further to expose this space. IVC should be further dissected medially to identify the left renal vein. Care should be taken in order to avoid avulsion of the lumbar veins which are located on the posterolateral aspect of the IVC. The renal artery is carefully dissected in this space. The renal vein now is skeletonized. Once again care should be taken to avoid bleeding from small branches. Once the hilar vessels are dissected, the lateral attachments are released, and the kidney is fully mobilized.

6.3   Retrieval of the Kidney

At this stage a 5–6 cm Pfannenstiel incision is made at the previously marked site. The anterior rectus fascia is incised and the upper and lower fascial layers are separated from the rectus muscle. The rectus is divided at midline and retracted laterally. The pre-peritoneal space is developed at the right side of the bladder and urachus without any breach of the peritoneal cavity. Under direct vision a 15 mm port is inserted which can be used to deploy the endovascular stapling device if the angles are appropriate. The length of this incision should be enough to easily accommodate surgeon's hand and the kidney including the Gerota's fascia.

Prior to advancing to the next stage, a series of checks should be performed.

1. The transplant surgeon should be scrubbed and acknowledge readiness to receive the kidney. Preservation fluid, ice slush, and back table instruments should all be available.
2. Open nephrectomy tray should be available and circulating nurse present in the room and ready.
3. The Anesthetist should be notified and muscle relaxation confirmed. An intravenous dose of mannitol should be given.
4. The laparoscopy tower checked for adequate insufflation gas.
5. Preloaded Hem-o-lok™ applicator and reload clips, vascular stapler, and a reload cartridge as well as the laparoscopic Satinsky clamp all available and within reach.

Following the final check, the kidney is once again inspected to ensure that there are no attachments except for the hilar vessels and the ureter. The ureter is now divided at the level of the pelvic brim (Figs. 6.13 and 6.14). Sucker tip is placed between the renal artery and vein to retract the kidney upward. Care should be taken to avoid excessive traction on hilar vessels. Prior to ligation and division of vessels, all steps should be mentally visualized. The renal artery is clipped with two Hem-o-lok™ clips (Fig. 6.15) as well as an additional titanium clip at the retrocaval region or the interaortocaval space as described previously. The artery is divided with a 2 mm cuff on the stay side. The warm ischemia time will start and should be recorded from application of the first clip. The laparoscopic staple device is now placed on the renal vein (Fig. 6.16), flushed to the IVC's lateral edge, and fired. The vein is cut above the last staple row (Fig. 6.17). The kidney is grasped by the forceps from the upper working port and handed to the assistant. The peritoneal layer of the Pfannenstiel incision is now opened, and the kidney is grasped by the surgeon's hand, retrieved, and subsequently handed over to the transplant surgeon for placement on ice slush and perfusion of the preservation fluid. While the transplant surgeon is attending to the kidney, the donor surgeon will need to reestablish pneumoperitoneum by placing a large sponge over the Pfannenstiel incision and inspect for major bleeding. At this stage, pneumoperitoneum can be slowly reduced

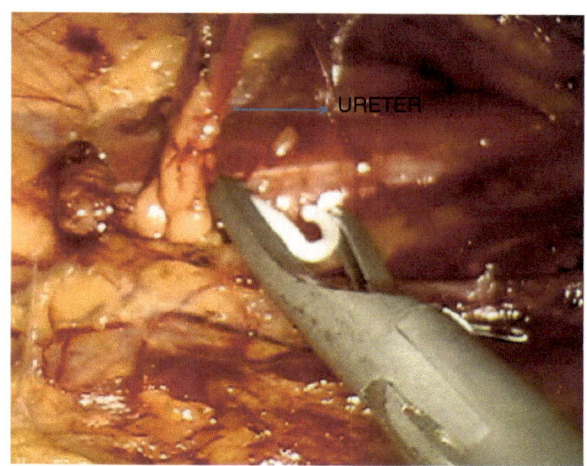

Fig. 6.13 Showing the ureter being clipped

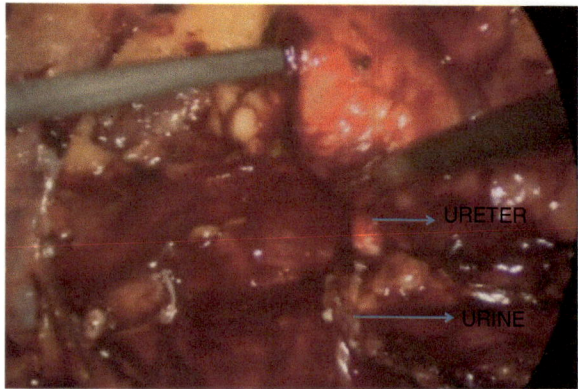

Fig. 6.14 Shows efflux of urine after the ureter is cut

Fig. 6.15 Shows clipped
renal artery

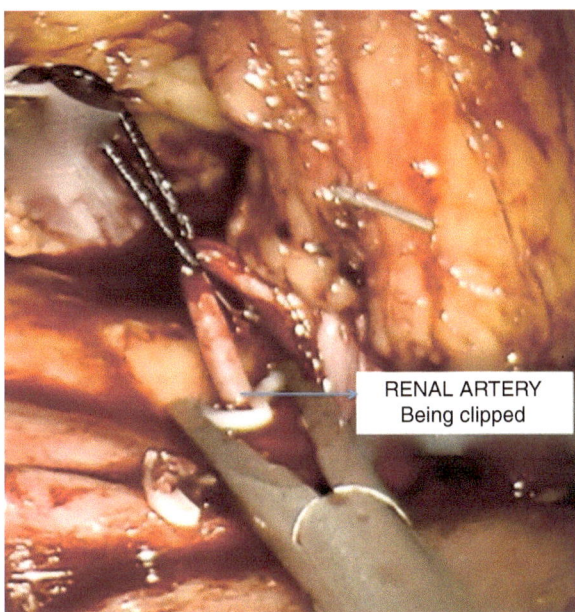

RENAL ARTERY
Being clipped

Fig. 6.16 Shows the renal
vein being stapled

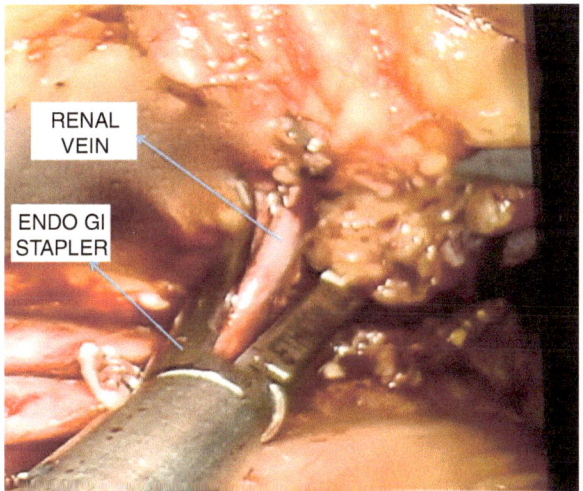

RENAL
VEIN

ENDO GI
STAPLER

to inspect for venous bleeding, which may have been tamponaded by the positive pressure of the pneumoperitoneum. If there is minor oozing from any site, hemostatic agents could be used. We usually do not put a drain unless significant oozing is encountered.

Local anesthetic is infiltrated in the surgical wounds. The peritoneal layer of the Pfannenstiel incision is closed with 3-0 Vicryl suture. The rectus muscles are gently approximated with 2-0 Vicryl sutures, and the anterior rectus fascia is closed with PDS sutures in a continuous manner. The 12 and 15 mm ports require fascial layer

Fig. 6.17 Shows stapled
renal vein

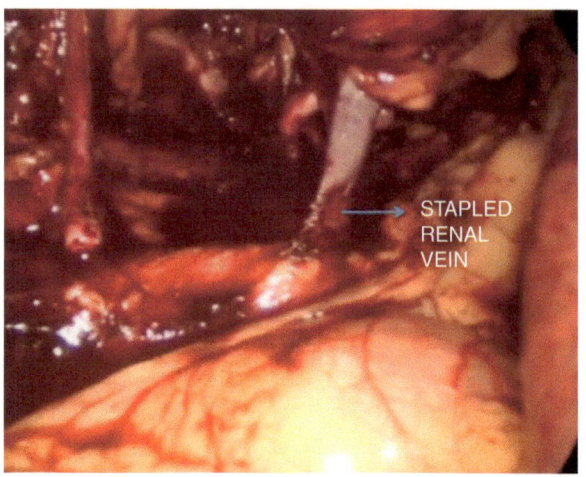

closures. The skin is closed with absorbable sutures to ensure maximum cosmetic
outcome for the donors.

Postoperative care of the donor patients includes diet as tolerated, supplemental
intravenous fluid, DVT prophylaxis with subcutaneous heparin, as well as early
mobilization. The urinary catheter is removed on the next day, and most patients are
able to be discharged within the first 2 days of the procedure. They will be subsequently followed up in clinic at 1 week and 6–8 weeks postoperatively.

References

1. Ratner LE, Ciseck LJ, Moore RG, Cigarroa FG, Kaufman HS, Kavoussi LR. Laparoscopic live
   donor nephrectomy. Transplantation. 1995;60(9):1047–9.
2. Abrahams HM, Freise CE, Kang SM, Stoller ML, Meng MV. Technique, indications and outcomes of pure laparoscopic right donor nephrectomy. J Urol. 2004;171(5):1793–6.
3. Afaneh C, Ramasamy R, Leeser DB, Kapur S, Del Pizzo JJ. Is right-sided laparoendoscopic
   single-site donor nephrectomy feasible? Urology. 2011;77(6):1365–9.
4. Jacobs SC, Cho E, Dunkin BJ, Flowers JL, Schweitzer E, Cangro C, et al. Laparoscopic live
   donor nephrectomy: the University of Maryland 3-year experience. J Urol.
   2000;164(5):1494–9.
5. Mandal AK, Cohen C, Montgomery RA, Kavoussi LR, Ratner LE. Should the indications for
   laparascopic live donor nephrectomy of the right kidney be the same as for the open procedure?
   Anomalous left renal vasculature is not a contraindiction to laparoscopic left donor nephrectomy. Transplantation. 2001;71(5):660–4.
6. Wang K, Zhang P, Xu X, Fan M. Right versus left laparoscopic living-donor nephrectomy: a
   meta-analysis. Exp Clin Transplant. 2015;13(3):214–26.

Hilar Control in Laparoscopic Donor Nephrectomy: Clips, Staplers and Other Methods

Ananthakrishnan Sivaraman, Abhishek Bhat, and Kulthe Ramesh Seetharam Bhat

Abstract

Laparoscopic donor nephrectomy (LDN) is today considered the standard of care for live kidney harvest in transplantations. Generally those who are considered fit for an open donor nephrectomy will be able to withstand the surgery by laparoscopy. Traditionally right-sided donor kidney, multiple vessels, vessel anomalies and obesity have been considered as relative contraindications; however, with growing skills and practices, they have been rendered obsolete. In this chapter, we emphasize on the different methods of hilar control. We highlight the techniques, difficulties in hilar control and ways to increase the vein length particularly on the right side.

7.1   Introduction

Laparoscopic donor nephrectomy (LDN) is today considered the standard of care for live kidney harvest in transplantations. Generally those who are considered fit for an open donor nephrectomy will be able to withstand the surgery by laparoscopy. Traditionally right-sided donor kidney, multiple vessels, vessel anomalies and obesity have been considered as relative contraindications; however, with growing skills and practices, they have been rendered obsolete. In this chapter, we emphasize on the different methods of hilar control. We highlight the techniques, difficulties in hilar control and ways to increase the vein length particularly on the right side.

A. Sivaraman (✉) • A. Bhat • K.R.S. Bhat
Department of Urology & Robotic Surgery, Apollo Hospitals, Chennai, India
e-mail: ananthsiv@gmail.com

© Springer Nature Singapore Pte Ltd. 2017
M.R. Desai, A.P. Ganpule (eds.), *Laparoscopic Donor Nephrectomy*,
DOI 10.1007/978-981-10-2849-6_7

7.2   Technique and Difficulties with Hilar Control and Techniques to Increase Renal Vein Length in Laparoscopic Donor Nephrectomy (LLDN)

The procedure of LDN has undergone many developmental stages at transplant centres across the globe, and many alterations have been practised to better donor and recipient outcomes. LDN is unique as this procedure involves a fit individual who has a major organ removed for the benefit of another. There is an overall perception in the transplant fraternity that this surgery is fairly safe. The most challenging and interesting step during laparoscopic donor nephrectomy is control of the pedicle [1].

Although previously of limited practice, right laparoscopic donor nephrectomy is becoming increasingly popular when left nephrectomy is not indicated [2]. LDN can be done either transperitoneal or retroperitoneal on either side, with transperitoneal being favoured by more institutions worldwide. The vessels are sequentially clipped and divided using Weck clips or ligated using the Endo GIA stapler and extracted via a Pfannenstiel incision. The pneumoperitoneum is reduced to minimum to confirm haemostasis before closure.

The variation on the right side lies in the requirement of an additional port which allows the Endo GIA stapler placement, allowing preservation of maximum length of the vein, by taking control at the renal vein – inferior vena caval junction [3]. Several modifications exist for increasing the length of the renal vein. The first method uses a TA stapler that can fire two lines of staple without cutting. To attain further length, the vein is then cut close to the staple line. The stapler is inserted through the lateral port, in a parallel to the inferior vena cava. The matching direction of the stapler with the IVC results in achieving the additional length on the right renal vein [2]. Second modification is to divide the right renal vein using a small subcostal incision on the right side after mobilizing the right kidney laparoscopically and placing a Satinsky clamp on the IVC, just medial to the origin of the renal vein. A laparoscopic Satinsky clamp may be needed to gain a cuff of IVC, which is subsequently sutured intracorporeally [4]. Third description is the use of the saphenous vein from the recipient when the renal vein is short for reconstruction and lengthening the renal vein.

7.3   Available Options for Hilar Control

To control the renal hilum, several options exist for the laparoscopic donor surgeon. Approximately 70% of the reported centres make use of the stapler on the renal artery; centres universally use this device on the renal vein. Hem-o-lok® clip may help gain additional length on the renal artery by sidestepping clips or staples on the side of the graft, and 28% of centres reported the use of this method. The possible alternatives are suture ligature, over sewing or stapling. Techniques that utilize vessel transfixation are technically arduous, time-consuming and challenging [7].

7.4 Clips

The traditional usage of clips has been perceived with a degree of doubt, owing to the reported deaths secondary to postoperative haemorrhage, following LDN since 2005, attributable to insecure renal artery ligation. This was followed by a safety information warning by US FDA in 2011, informing that Hem-o-lok clips are contraindicated in ligation of the renal artery in LDN. Recent reports concerning vascular clips becoming dislodged or tearing vessels leading to haemorrhage and even death raise serious concerns about their use in LDN.

Although the package inserts for specific devices caution the use on major vessels, many surgeons do not strictly observe instructions from the manufacturer of these devices. Explanations for this include that the unexpected situations in surgeries occur less frequently, the development of new applications for devices intended for specific use and the natural ingenuity which many innovative surgeons apply to the advantage of their patients every day. However, at least one specific device should not be applied on the renal artery as there were at least 13 complications due to this or a similar device, with all but one complication detected in the late intraoperative or postoperative period. Therefore, the package inserts are not necessarily wrong in contraindicating the use of these for primary renal artery control. Locking clips also did not have any safety benefit as arterial haemorrhage were seen in eight patients in either the late intraoperative or postoperative time period [5]. However, this must be balanced with the view that for most laparoscopic and robotic radical nephrectomies, the Hem-o-lok clips seem to be of standard usage. Given that the number of radical nephrectomies is far more common than the donor nephrectomies, we urge the individual departments to take a consensus opinion on the usage of hem-o-lok clips.

Most surgeons employ polymer or titanium clips for arterial control and the Endo GIA stapler for the vein. However, this stapler is also prone for misfire and is not cost-effective. [8]. A 1-mm vascular cuff augments the safety of both the non absorbable polymer ligating (NPL) and titanium clips in all-sized blood vessels. NPL clip was statistically safer on 10-mm cuffed and uncuffed vessels and 6-mm cuffed arteries than the titanium clip. The NPL clip is steadfast and dependable in securing both arteries and veins [8]. Moreover, in the senior author's experience, the traction to the kidney, applied while applying clips during laparoscopic donor nephrectomy in order to gain length in the artery, has a negative effect like intimal tears as well as clip slippage due to tenting of the renal artery at the origin of the aorta. Hence, traction should be reduced during clip application.

Usage of the Endo GIA stapler for the hilum has substantial cost burden in comparison with only Hem-o-lok clips. The cost of a single Hem-o-lok clip cartridge with six clips is about 20 euros, and the additional expenses of sterilizing the clip applicator are little, while the disposable Endo GIA stapler with two clip cartridges necessary for both the artery and vein is 245 euros [6].

Hem-o-lok technique is quicker than applying the Endo GIA, and the whole procedure of dissection, ligation and division can be done within 10 min. It is technically simpler than using the Endo GIA, especially in the retroperitoneum with limited space when the kidney is approached retroperitoneally [6].

Hem-o-lok clips permitted a substantial length of the renal vein to be removed during LDN since the applicator is not bulky and less problematic to apply over the vein when compared to the Endo GIA. A supplementary advantage of the Hem-o-lok clip is that it can be introduced via a 10-mm port, but a 12-mm port is compulsory for the other, and its usage was found to be accompanied with less tremor, the reason being probably the fact that the Endo GIA has a 5-mm stem through the larger port [7].

Intraoperative clip malfunction is not infrequent. Two cases of perioperative clip dysfunction during laparoscopic donor nephrectomy with the techniques to control them have been described. In one such case of left-hand-assisted LDN, the clips placed on the renal artery slipped, and the surgeon compressed the source of bleeding using his finger following which an occlusion balloon catheter was introduced through the femoral artery and advanced to the origin of the renal artery. With the control of haemorrhage, the renal artery stump was repaired by laparoscopic suturing, thus avoiding conversion to open. In the second incident, the stump length was long enough for clips to be placed again [8].

Elliot et al. studied the bursting pressures in various procedures of renal artery control and probable failure mechanism on porcine models. The mean bursting pressures for the clips were found to be higher than the normal arterial pressures (1220–1500 mmHg). But the vessels closed with the stapler had leak at low pressure (262 mmHg). Retraction of the vessel into and behind the clip was the reason for bleeding when titanium or the self-locking polymer clips were used, while it occurred in between the individual staples in the staple line. The number of clips or the stump length did not affect the bursting pressures with the titanium or polymer clips. It was consequently concluded that improved safety was not guaranteed with the traditional measures of additional cuff length or clips [9].

Kapoor et al. reported in 246 laparoscopic nephrectomies with arterial and venous control obtained via Hem-o-lok clips only (2 on the patient side). There were no cases of reported blood transfusion attributable to clip failure [10].

7.5   Staplers

The complication rate of around 2% exists when using staplers for renal vein ligations, which are complications like open conversion (20–27%) and blood transfusion (15%). The main reasons of associated complications are due to poor technique of instrumentation or due to the use of staples with incorrect width. For an adequate positioning of staple before ligation, at least 3 cm of the vein should be dissected, to reduce complication rates. This is relatively tedious on the right

Fig. 7.1 Hem-o-lok™ clips. The cardinal rules for application of these clips are as follows: (1) The knob of the clip should be seen. (2) The click of the clip should be heard. (3) The vessel to be clipped should be circumferentially dissected. (4) Two clips should be applied always on the patient side. (5) A cuff of 2 mm should be kept beyond the clip

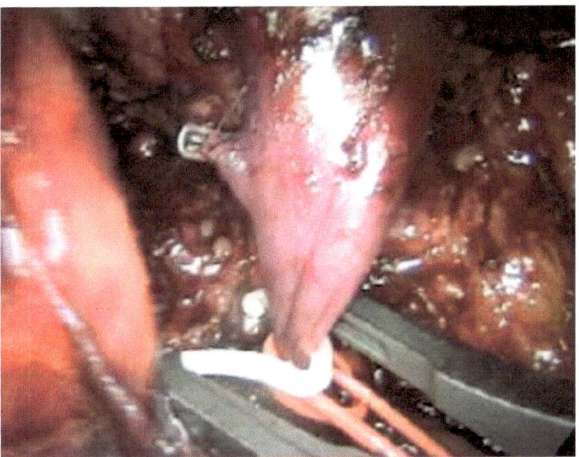

side particularly due to short renal vein. It must be ensured that earlier positioned clips used for the three tributaries should be avoided on the left side, as it may hinder the proper application of the Endo GIA stapler by getting trapped between the jaws of the stapler. Only about less than 0.3 and 0.5% have been found to primarily malfunction [11].

Ryan SA Hsi et al. reported a review on failure to describe the mechanisms of clip and stapler failure during LDN. Ninety-two cases of complications due to device malfunction were identified, out of which 59 (64%) were due to endoscopic stapler failure, 21 (23%) due to titanium clip failure and 12 (13%) due to locking clip failure. The most common mechanisms for failure of stapler were either missed or poorly formed stapler lines (51%) and failed stapler release (25%). The most common titanium clip-related failures were due to scissoring or disfigurement of clips (52%), jamming (19%) and slippage (14%). It is estimated that the overall failure rate for titanium clips was about 4.9%, about 3% for staplers and about 1.9% while using locking clips [12].

Though the endovascular GIA staplers are convenient during laparoscopic nephrectomy, it may malfunction leading to substantial blood loss and consequent open conversion. Most problems could be circumvented with diligent application and early detection [11].

Ko et al. in their 10-year analysis of laparoscopic donor nephrectomy programme of 400 cases reported four stapler-related dysfunctions; all were on the left side, two of which had to be converted to open to attain haemostasis. It was concluded that the Endo GIA stapler is safe for both the left and right LDN. Endo GIA stapler has now standardized the procedure, thus reducing the need for supplementary manoeuvres in safeguarding the renal hilum, meanwhile producing similar outcomes [9] (Figs. 7.1 and 7.2).

Fig. 7.2 The staplers should be applied only in completely dissected vessels

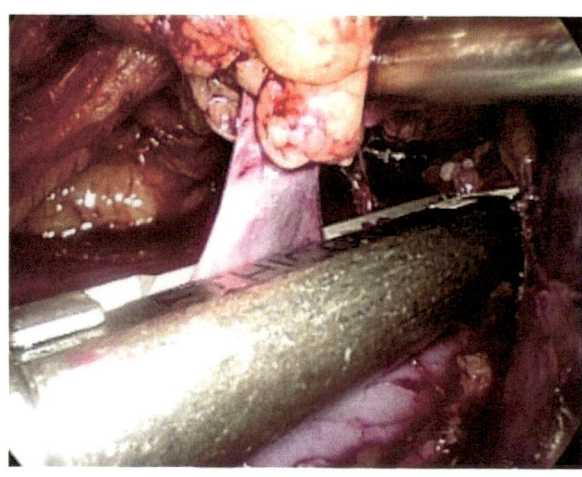

7.6   Other Alternatives for Hilar Control

Numerous substitutes for renal vein ligation other than the Endo GIA stapler have been described while developing laparoscopic nephrectomy. Kadirkamanathan described the placement of knots on the renal hilar vessels intracorporeally [13]. Ultrasonic scalpel and bipolar device have been tried on a porcine model successfully [14]. Nevertheless, these techniques were deemed to be unpredictable.

Janetschek et al. described a technique of extracorporeal knots to reduce its diameter prior to the application of Hem-o-lok clips and effectively used this technique for 20 nephrectomies [15]. A knot pusher was used to push the knot down around the renal vein, although this was accomplished with precision to avoid any injury to the vein. On an average, 2 min was needed for placing knots, thus preventing its application during LDN to reduce the warm ischaemia time. Lately, modifications to this technique included manual constriction of the renal vein before the application of Hem-o-lok clip [16].

Numerous variations have been proposed to easily and safely harvest the right kidney via laparoscopic approach. Gill et al. have reported right-sided donor nephrectomy via retroperitoneoscopy. An Endo GIA stapler was used for dividing the renal vessels following which bench dissection was performed to free the hilar vessels, thus gaining additional length for the vascular anastomosis [17]. Lee et al. described a laparoscopic-assisted technique where a horizontal incision of 8 cm was placed in the upper quadrant on the right side which was used to pass a Satinsky clamp over the IVC, and the same was used for vessel control, kidney extraction and repair of cavotomy [18].

A modified Satinsky atraumatic vascular clamp, intended for thoracoscopic procedures, has been used for the purpose of right-sided nephrectomies

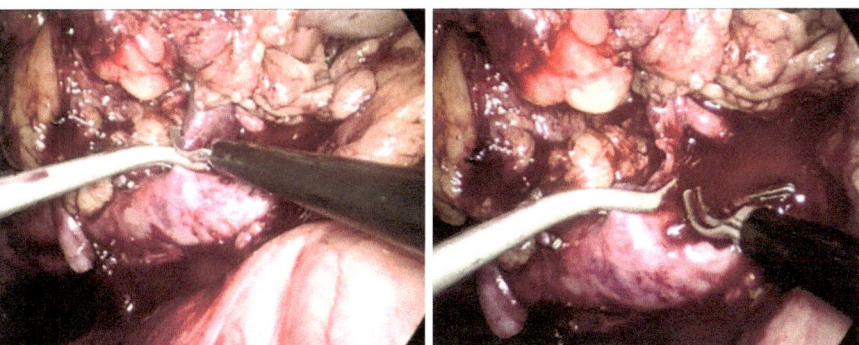

Fig. 7.3 Satinsky clamp

Fig. 7.4 The application
of the Satinsky clamp
helps in gaining vein
length. The vein length is
gained by procuring the
cuff of the vena cava

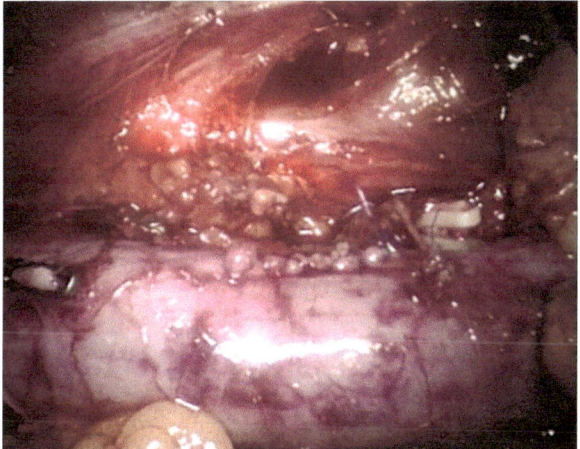

(Figs. 7.3 and 7.4). A tiny incision is placed to the right side of the anterior superior
iliac spine and is used to clamp the IVC and divide the adjacent renal vein with scissors. This modified instrument is longer than the routine clamp and is inserted without trocar into the peritoneum. The IVC is sutured laparoscopically with 3-0 running
PDS suture prior to the clamp removal. Also, Scandinavian surgeons sidestep difficult anastomosis due to short renal vein by dividing the internal iliac vein, thus
helping them to deliver the external iliac veins to the superficial wound, thus speed-
ing up the anastomosis [4].

Regardless of the method of vascular control employed, the major vessels should
be dissected all around, prior to securing them (Fig. 7.5).

Fig. 7.5 Whichever
method of vascular control
is employed, the vessels
should be circumferentially
dissected prior to securing
them

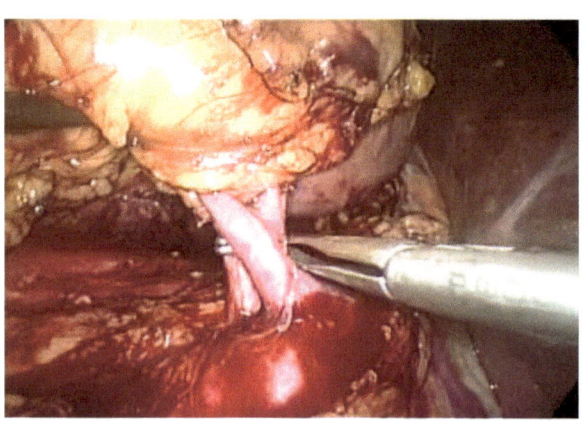

Conclusions

Laparoscopic donor nephrectomy is the preferred mode of renal procurement, and it demands more surgical skill compared to conventional open donor nephrectomy. The need for adequate length of the renal artery on the left side forces the surgeon to use a short renal artery stump. The need for securing the gonadal, lumbar and adrenal venous tributaries makes the situation difficult. The right side poses a problem with the short length of the renal vein.

Nonlocking polymer clips, locking clips, vascular staples and ligatures are utilized in today's scenario by different institutes, but none of them are considered foolproof. Stapling devices pose probability for missing or malformed staple lines and failure to release. In early branching renal arteries, surgeons find it technically challenging to get multiple renal arteries with graft rather than get the proximal end with single stem. Stapler and NPL are far more expensive than titanium clips. NPL clips increase the graft length; locking mechanism increases security. Titanium clips pose the risk of scissoring, malformation, jamming and dislodgement [19].

It is now decisively established that surgeons must be conversant with and foresee the likely issues that might crop up with all the techniques employed to control the renal hilum. Know-how of the probable device malfunction which is identified and necessary response can limit the morbidity of donor if they occur. Finally, it is the responsibility of the donor surgeon to advocate safe practices and actively participate in the manufacturing process for constant improvement of the safety of present devices [12].

References

1. Matas AJ, Payne WD, Sutherland DE, Humar A, Gruessner RW, Kandaswamy R, et al. 2,500 living donor kidney transplants: a single-center experience. Ann Surg. 2001;234(2):149–64.
2. Mendoza D, Newman RC, Albala D, Cohen MS, Tewari A, Lingeman J, et al. Laparoscopic complications in markedly obese urologic patients (a multi-institutional review). Urology. 1996;48(4):562–7.

3. Gupta N, Raina P, Kumar A. Laparoscopic donor nephrectomy. J Minim Access Surg. 2005;1(4):155–64.
4. Turk IA, Deger S, Davis JW, Giesing M, Fabrizio MD, Schönberger B, et al. Laparoscopic live donor right nephrectomy: a new technique with preservation of vascular length. J Urol. 2002;167(2 Pt 1):630–3.
5. Friedman AL, Peters TG, Jones KW, Boulware LE, Ratner LE. Fatal and nonfatal hemorrhagic complications of living kidney donation. Ann Surg. 2006;243(1):126–30.
6. Baumert H, Ballaro A, Arroyo C, Kaisary AV, Mulders PFA, Knipscheer BC. The use of polymer (Hem-o-lok) clips for management of the renal hilum during laparoscopic nephrectomy. Eur Urol. 2006;49(5):816–9.
7. Chueh S-CJ, Wang S-M, Lai M-K. Use of Hem-o-lok clips effectively lengthens renal vein during laparoscopic live donor nephrectomy. Transplant Proc. 2004;36(9):2623–4.
8. Maartense S, Heintjes RJ, Idu M, Bemelman FJ, Bemelman WA. Renal artery clip dislodgement during hand-assisted laparoscopic living donor nephrectomy. Surg Endosc. 2003; 17(11):1851.
9. Ko EY, Castle EP, Desai PJ, Moss AA, Reddy KS, Mekeel KL, et al. Utility of the endovascular stapler for right-sided laparoscopic donor nephrectomy: a 7-year experience at Mayo Clinic. J Am Coll Surg. 2008;207(6):896–903.
10. Kapoor R, Singh KJ, Suri A, Dubey D, Mandhani A, Srivastava A, et al. Hem-o-lok clips for vascular control during laparoscopic ablative nephrectomy: a single-center experience. J Endourol. 2006;20(3):202–4.
11. Chan D, Bishoff JT, Ratner L, Kavoussi LR, Jarrett TW. Endovascular gastrointestinal stapler device malfunction during laparoscopic nephrectomy: early recognition and management. J Urol. 2000;164(2):319–21.
12. Hsi RS, Ojogho ON, Baldwin DD. Analysis of techniques to secure the renal hilum during laparoscopic donor nephrectomy: review of the FDA database. Urology. 2009;74(1):142–7.
13. Kadirkamanathan SS, Shelton JC, Hepworth CC, Laufer JG, Swain CP. A comparison of the strength of knots tied by hand and at laparoscopy. J Am Coll Surg. 1996;182(1):46–54.
14. Landman J, Kerbl K, Rehman J, Andreoni C, Humphrey PA, Collyer W, et al. Evaluation of a vessel sealing system, bipolar electrosurgery, harmonic scalpel, titanium clips, endoscopic gastrointestinal anastomosis vascular staples and sutures for arterial and venous ligation in a porcine model. J Urol. 2003;169(2):697–700.
15. Janetschek G, Bagheri F, Abdelmaksoud A, Biyani CS, Leeb K, Jeschke S. Ligation of the renal vein during laparoscopic nephrectomy: an effective and reliable method to replace vascular staplers. J Urol. 2003;170(4 Pt 1):1295–7.
16. Eswar C, Badillo FL. Vascular control of the renal pedicle using the hem-o-lok polymer ligating clip in 50 consecutive hand-assisted laparoscopic nephrectomies. J Endourol. 2004;18(5): 459–61.
17. Gill IS, Uzzo RG, Hobart MG, Streem SB, Goldfarb DA, Noble MJ. Laparoscopic retroperitoneal live donor right nephrectomy for purposes of allotransplantation and autotransplantation. J Urol. 2000;164(5):1500–4.
18. Lee BR, Chow GK, Ratner LE, Kavoussi LR. Laparoscopic live donor nephrectomy: outcomes equivalent to open surgery. J Endourol. 2000;14(10):811. -819–820.
19. Kurukkal SN. Techniques to Secure Renal Hilum in Laparoscopic Donor Nephrectomy - REVIEW ARTICLES. World J Laparosc Surg SE - [Internet]. 2012; Available from: http:// dx.doi.org/10.5005/jp-journals-10007-1143.

Retroperitoneoscopic Donor Nephrectomy

8

S.J. Rizvi and P.R. Modi

Abstract

Since the first living-related kidney transplant in 1965, removal of the donated kidney was done by an open operation [1, 2]. Ways to minimise the morbidity of access included video-assisted mini-incision donor nephrectomy [3]. Laparoscopic donor nephrectomy (LDN) was first described by Ratner et al. in 1995 [4] and was accomplished by the transperitoneal route. This operation can be done by transperitoneal or retroperitoneal route. In this chapter we allude to the nuaces of port placement, dissection and troubleshooting in retroperitoneoscopic donor nephrectomy.

8.1 Introduction

Since the first living-related kidney transplant in 1965, removal of the donated kidney was done by an open operation [1, 2]. Ways to minimise the morbidity of access included video-assisted mini-incision donor nephrectomy [3]. Laparoscopic donor nephrectomy (LDN) was first described by Ratner et al. in 1995 [4] and was accomplished by the transperitoneal route. In the last two decades, this procedure has come to be considered the standard of care for living kidney donation. However like

S.J. Rizvi
Institute of Kidney Diseases and Research Center, Civil Hospital Campus, Aswara, Ahmedabad, India

P.R. Modi (✉)
Department of Transplantation Surgery and Urology, Smt. G. R. Doshi and Smt. K. M. Mehta Institute of Kidney Diseases and Research Centre & Dr. H. L. Trivedi Institute of Transplantation Sciences, Civil Hospital Campus, Asarwa, Ahmedabad, Gujarat, India
e-mail: dr_pranjal@yahoo.com

© Springer Nature Singapore Pte Ltd. 2017   83
M.R. Desai, A.P. Ganpule (eds.), *Laparoscopic Donor Nephrectomy*,
DOI 10.1007/978-981-10-2849-6_8

any other surgical operation, LDN has associated morbidity and mortality. This is of particular concern as the operation is performed on a normal individual motivated by altruistic considerations.

Thus there is a constant effort to look for refinements of technique that can result in greater patient safety and comfort while ensuring optimum graft retrieval. Hand-assisted retroperitoneoscopic donor nephrectomy was described as a way to provide minimal access while avoiding entering the peritoneal cavity and its potential sequelae [5–7]. It has been described as a useful technique in centres with limited experience of laparoscopy and retroperitoneoscopy. Mini-incision donor nephrectomy has been described in an attempt to minimise morbidity of access while maintaining donor safety [8].

In 1992 Gaur described retroperitoneal laparoscopic surgery [9]. The first retroperitoneal laparoscopic donor nephrectomy (RLDN) was described in 2000 by Gill [10], following demonstration of feasibility in a porcine model. It is not used as widely as transperitoneal laparoscopic donor nephrectomy, probably because of unfamiliarity with retroperitoneoscopy. RLDN gives quick and direct access to the renal vasculature. The lumbar vessels on the left side are excellently visualised. There is no manipulation of intra-abdominal viscera; this results in less postoperative pain and ileus in the short term and a reduced risk of complications related to adhesions in the long term. The risk of iatrogenic bowel injury is minimised. Postoperative collections of blood, lymph or chyle are localised and easier to manage.

Indications and contraindications: RLDN may be considered for nearly every living kidney donor. Retroperitoneoscopy is technically challenging in patients who have had prior open renal surgery; however it would be unusual for such an individual to be a kidney donor. Donors with all arterial and venous anomalies can be optimally managed with RLDN, as it provides excellent exposure to the vessels. The decision to accept a donor with vascular anomalies depends on the experience of the operating team. There are few if any contraindications to RLDN.

Preoperative preparation: Standard institutional protocol includes hemogram, kidney and liver function tests, urinalysis, lymphocyte crossmatch and single antigen test to detect donor-specific antibodies. We perform a nuclear renal scan for differential renal function and a CT renal angiography with CT IVP to delineate donor arterial, venous and collecting system anatomy. High BMI individuals are encouraged to lose weight prior to donation. Donors with conditions such as hypertension, obesity, stone disease, etc. are taken in accordance with the Amsterdam guidelines [11].

Side selection: The left kidney is preferred in view of the longer left renal vein. The right kidney is selected for reasons such as multiple left-sided renal arteries, differential renal function favouring the left kidney or pathology such as cysts or calculi affecting the right kidney.

Perioperative management: Donors are hydrated overnight with intravenous fluids. Compression stockings are applied prior to positioning to reduce the risk of deep vein thrombosis and pulmonary embolism. Intraoperatively circulating volume is maintained with crystalloid and colloid solutions. IV mannitol is given intraoperatively. We do not heparinise the donor prior to control of the renal artery.

Armamentarium: No special surgical or laparoscopic instruments are required. Small cat's paw retractors are useful for creation of the first port. Proprietary energy sources such as LigaSure™, Harmonic Scalpel™ or Thunderbeat™ are useful adjuncts.

Checklist of instruments:

For retroperitoneal access:
    Small right-angled retractors
    Blunt gauze dissector (peanut)
    Balloon
Laparoscopic instruments (5 mm)
    Five and 10 mm ports
    Blunt suction
    Laparoscopic hook
    Maryland forceps
    Blunt-tipped forceps
    Right-angled forceps
    Scissors
    Five and 10 mm polymer clip applicators
Energy sources
    Monopolar electrocautery
    Bipolar electrocautery
    Ultrasonic energy (e.g. Harmonic Scalpel®)
    Bipolar sealing devices (e.g. LigaSure®, Thunderbeat®)

Balloon: The indigenously made balloon as described by Gaur is cost-effective and efficacious. It consists of a 12 Fr. plastic catheter with two fingers of a size 8 surgical glove securely tied to the end using silk ties (Fig. 8.1). In our experience we

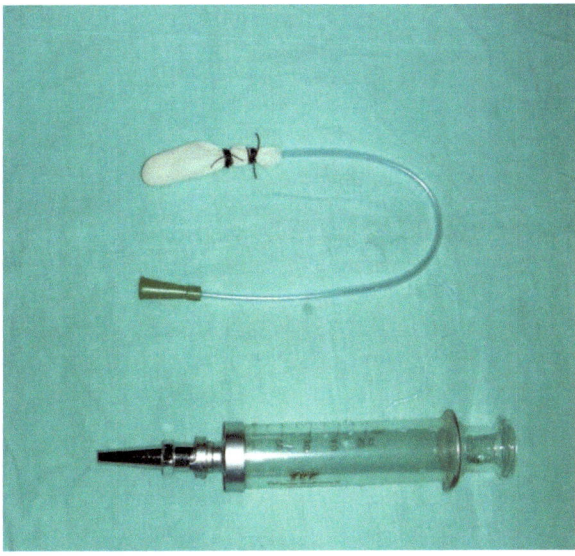

Fig. 8.1 Indigenously made balloon with syringe for inflation

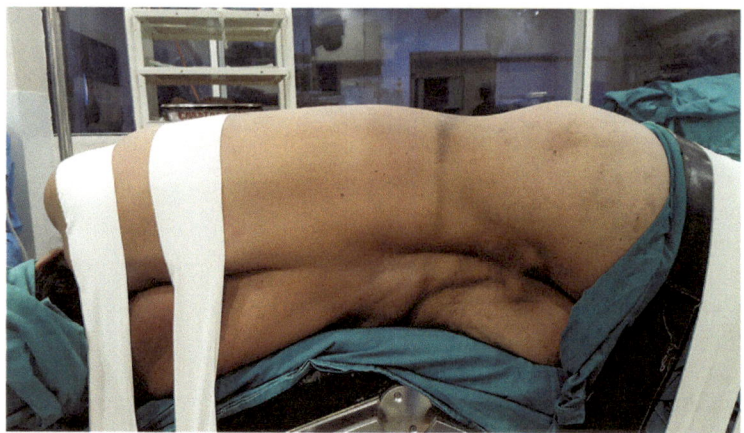

Fig. 8.2 Position for right RLDN

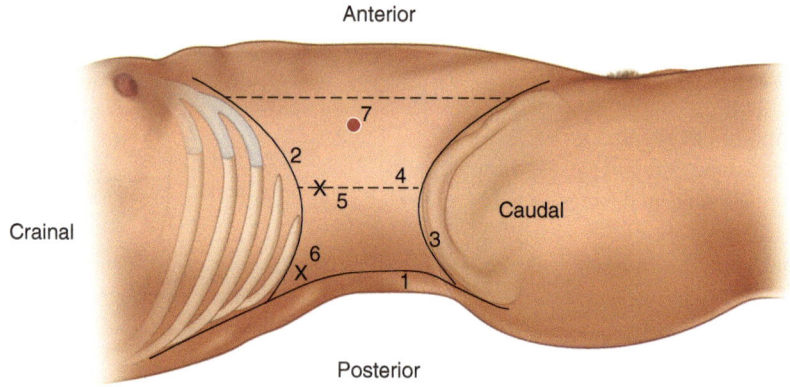

Fig. 8.3 Port placement for right RLDN

have never had failure of retroperitoneal access due to balloon malfunction. A variety of commercially manufactured balloons are available and may be used.

Steps for left RLDN. Differences for right-sided procedure are described subsequently.

Position: The patient is catheterised and placed in a standard flank position on the edge of the operating table. The flank muscles are placed on stretch by breaking the table or using a bridge (Fig. 8.2). Secure fixation is achieved by using adhesive tape or broad straps. The patient is draped to include the tenth rib and the ipsilateral groin in the operative field.

Port placement: Port placement (Fig. 8.3).

The landmarks are as follows:

1. Paraspinous muscles
2. Costal margin

Fig. 8.4 Creation of first port

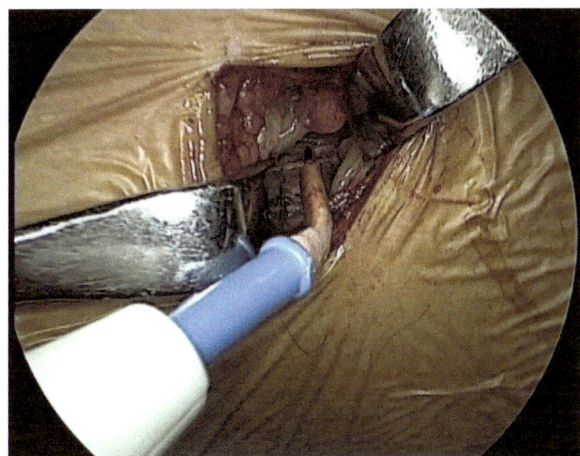

3. Iliac crest
4. Mid-axillary line

   Port sites:

5. First port (10 mm): 1 cm below intersection of costal margin and mid-axillary line
6. Second port (10 mm): renal angle, at least three fingerbreadths distant from first port
7. Third port (5 mm): three fingerbreadths anterior to first port, forming a straight line with the other ports

STEPS: Open access to the retroperitoneum is carried out by placing a 1.5 cm incision. The lumbodorsal fascia is similarly incised, allowing the paranephric fat to be seen. Craniocaudal movement to the paranephric fat with respiration aids in its identification. A peanut is used to sweep the Gerota's fascia and its contents anteriorly off the psoas muscle, to create space for a balloon. The balloon is inserted in the retroperitoneum and inflated with saline to create the retroperitoneal space. About 500 ml of saline is used. A palpable lump confirms the extraperitoneal situation of the balloon. The balloon is then deflated and removed and must be visually inspected to ensure intactness (Fig. 8.4).

Fixation sutures of no.1 silk are taken, preferable incorporating some of the muscular fascia. However this might be difficult in an obese donor and may be omitted. The port is inserted and insufflation with CO_2 started. The 10 mm laparoscope is then inserted into the retroperitoneum and intactness of peritoneum confirmed. The scope is withdrawn 1 cm into the port and the port withdrawn until the fascial edges are visualised and then slightly advanced until the edges are no longer seen. This ensures that the inner end of the port is at the edge of the operative field and maximises the visual field. The port is then fixed by securely tying the fixing sutures around it. This step is unnecessary if using self-retaining ports. The laparoscope is inserted and rotated to the 30 ° up position to view the abdominal wall anterior to it. The reflected edge of the peritoneum should be looked for, and digital pressure on the site of the second port should confirm that the site of entry is posterior to the peritoneal reflection (Fig. 8.5); a 5 mm port is inserted and fixed securely. The vision is now directed posteriorly and inferiorly and the site confirmed by digitally indenting the skin over the renal angle. Overlying adherent paranephric fat or Gerota's fascia may be swept away using blunt or sharp dissection with an instrument inserted through the second port. A 10 mm port is inserted. The insufflation tube is shifted to this port and pneumoperitoneum maintained at 12–15 mmHg.

Landmarks: The major landmark in retroperitoneal laparoscopy is the psoas muscle (Fig. 8.6). This should be prominently seen and kept in a horizontal orientation at all times. Gerota's fascia is seen anterior to the psoas muscle, although it may

Fig. 8.5 Insertion of second port showing peritoneal reflection

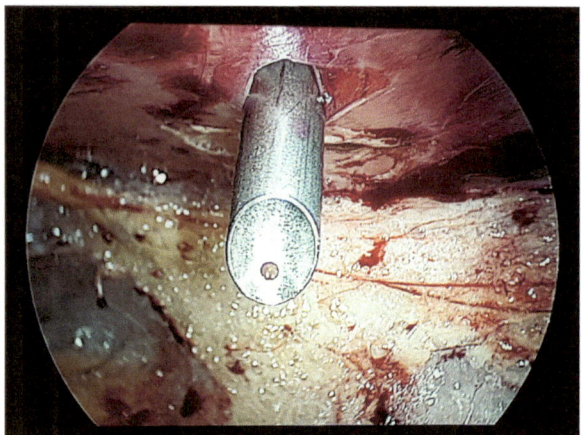

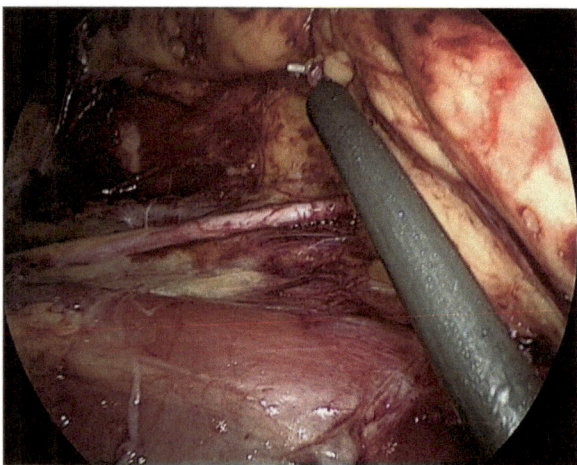

Fig. 8.6 The psoas muscle is the most important landmark in RLDN

be obscured by abundant paranephric fat. Anterior to this the peritoneal reflection is seen. Using an energy source, the Gerota's fascia is incised from the mid-ureter to the upper pole of the kidney, close to the psoas muscle (Fig. 8.7). This brings the perinephric fat, ureter and tissue surrounding the renal hilum into view. The ureter is bluntly dissected, keeping the periureteric fascia intact. Energy may be used sparingly to control the segmental blood supply. It is not necessary to remove the gonadal vein along with the ureter.

The kidney is elevated using a blunt instrument in the 5 mm port, thus placing the renal hilum on stretch. Preservation of the posterior layer of perinephric fat cushions the renal parenchyma from injury due to the lifting instrument. Hook with electrocautery or bipolar energy is used to divide the fibro-lymphatic tissue overlying the renal hilum (Fig. 8.8). This step brings the renal vein with its tributaries and the renal artery into view. The pattern of renal vein tributaries on the left side is

Fig. 8.7 Incision of Gerota's fascia

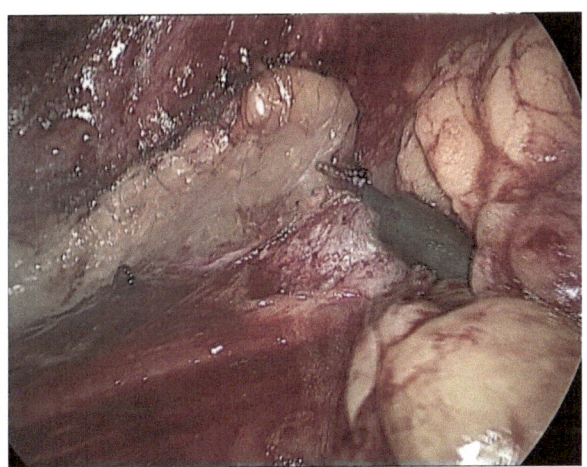

Fig. 8.8 Dissection of the renal hilum

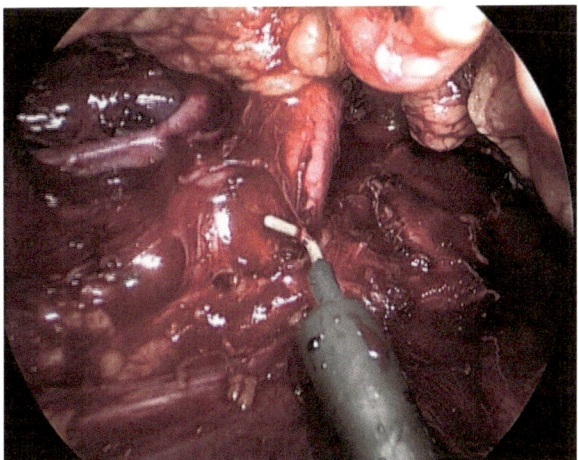

variable, and therefore the anatomy should be clearly delineated prior to division of any vessel. The lumbar vein is a posterior tributary of the renal vein and is often closely applied to the renal artery as it courses into the posterior abdominal wall (Fig. 8.9). Care should therefore be taken to achieve separation from the renal artery before application of energy. This vessel may be divided between 5 mm titanium or polymer clips or sealed and divided using energy sources such as LigaSure. The distal gonadal vein is traced until its confluence with the renal vein, where it may be controlled and divided or retained as a stay to keep the renal vein stretched and facilitate its dissection.

A combination of blunt and sharp dissection is used to bare the proximal renal artery and a few millimetres of the aorta surrounding its origin (Fig. 8.10). Great care should be taken to avoid thermal injury to the renal artery. The posterior layer of perinephric fat may be excised using hook electrocautery, thereby baring the

Fig. 8.9 Dissection of lumbar veins, showing the excellent access afforded by RLDN

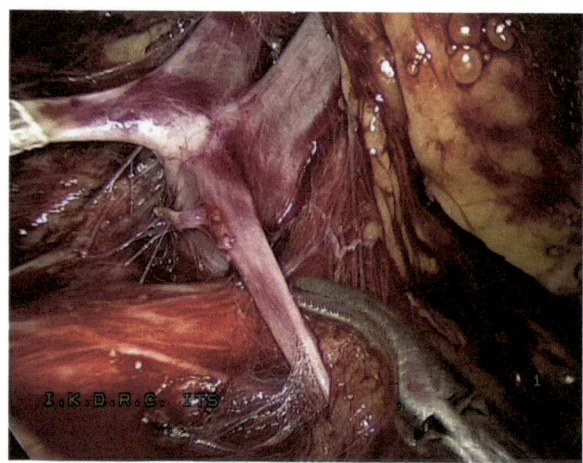

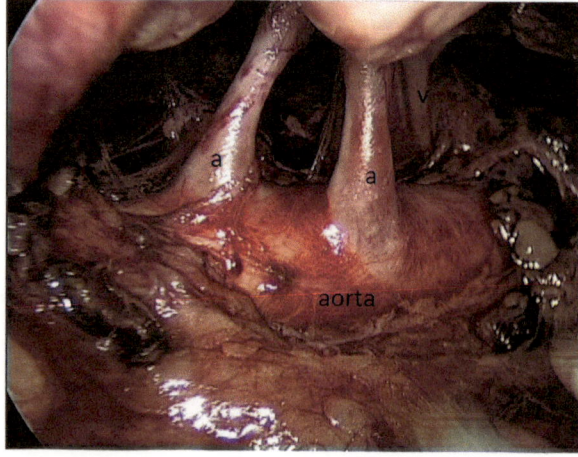

Fig. 8.10 Dissected renal artery and vein, in a donor with two renal arteries. *a* Artery, *v* vein

posterior surface of the kidney. The kidney is progressively mobilised from the upper to the lower pole anteriorly, and the kidney is pushed inferiorly and posteriorly. Care should be taken not to unduly stretch the renal artery. Vessels coursing towards the adrenal gland from the hilum should be controlled and divided. The renal vein can be dissected medially at this stage as the kidney is flipped posteriorly.

The lower pole is then flipped laterally and superiorly and dissection commenced in a plane between the periureteric fat and the peritoneum. Care must be taken to avoid injury to the ureter and peritoneum. This lateral displacement completes the mobilisation of the kidney and separation from the peritoneum. Any remaining attachments can be divided, including the gonadal vein if not previously done. The ureter is clipped as low as possible and divided using cold shears just proximal to the clip.

A 6–7 cm long incision is made about 1.5 cm superior and parallel to the inguinal ligament. The external oblique fascia is sharply divided and the transversus abdominis and internal oblique fibres split to expose the preperitoneal fat, which is kept intact to minimise loss of CO_2. The wound is packed with a wet mop to minimise gas loss.

The renal artery is first controlled with a stapler or two polymer clips [12] and divided with Endo Shears. When polymer clips are used, care must be taken to leave at least 2–3 mm stump of the renal artery beyond the clip. The artery must be dissected cleanly all around, and a distinct click sound should be heard at the time of application of the clip. The renal vein is then put on stretch and similarly controlled. Care should be taken during control of the renal vein not to dislodge clips on the arterial stump. Security can be augmented by using a combination of polymer and titanium clips [13]. The surgeon's left hand is then inserted into the extraction incision and the kidney retrieved, placed in ice slush and perfused.

The retrieval incision is closed in layers. Pneumoperitoneum is re-established and the retroperitoneum inspected for haemostasis and appropriate measures taken to control bleeding vessels. Inspection should be performed with a pneumoperitoneum of 5 mmHg to look for venous bleeding which could be tamponaded by higher gas pressures. It is our practice to clip large lymphatic tissue around the renal artery stump to minimise chances of lymphatic or chylous collections, which are a rare but serious complication of left donor nephrectomy. These vessels may sometimes by observed to ooze milky fluid. The second and third ports should be removed under vision. An attempt should be made to close the sheath of the camera port, but this may be difficult in individuals with abundant subcutaneous tissue and may be omitted. The skin is closed with Monocryl subcuticular sutures.

8.2   Modifications for Right-Sided RDN

Additional port: 12 mm port is placed 1 cm superior to the iliac crest and 1 cm posterior to the mid-axillary line (Fig. 8.11). Dissection proceeds in a manner similar to the left-sided nephrectomy. The gonadal vein should be identified till its confluence with the IVC and separated from the ureter to minimise chances of avulsion. The renal artery can be dissected for a considerable distance posterior to the IVC. The renal vein is dissected,

Fig. 8.11 Placement of fourth port in right-sided RLDN

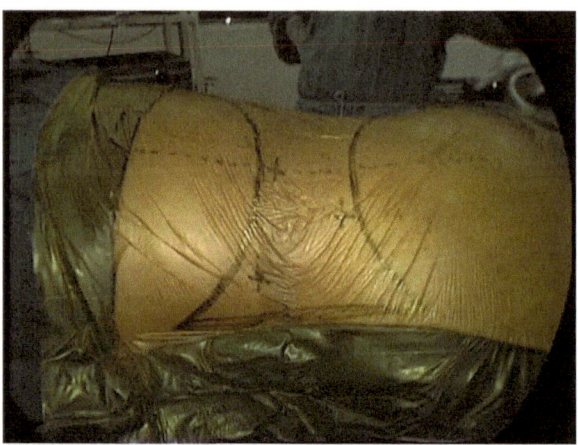

Fig. 8.12 Tenting of the IVC prior to applying the stapler on the right renal vein

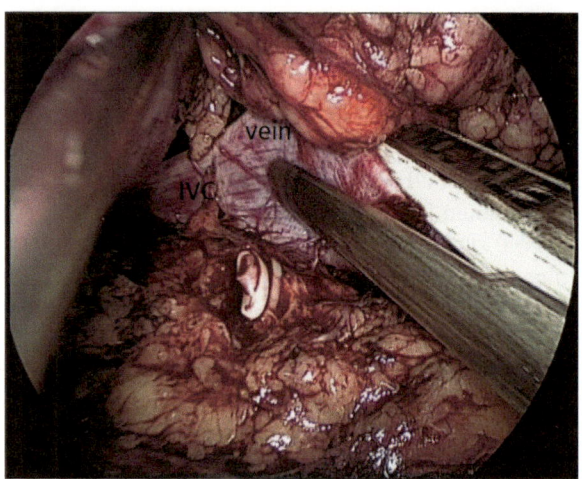

clearing the IVC around its confluence, and for a few centimetres in a cephalic direction to allow the tented caval wall to be pulled up into the stapler. After division of the artery, a laparoscopic TA stapler is passed through the 12 mm port. The kidney is elevated to put the renal vein on stretch, and the stapler fired as low on the vein as possible, incorporating a cuff of IVC in the staple line [14] (Fig. 8.12). The stapler is removed and Endo Shears used to divide the tissue on the graft side of the staple line.

8.3   Troubleshooting

Obesity leading to difficulty in accurate creation of first port: Sometimes abundant subcutaneous fat can make it difficult to create a small incision in the flank muscles. In this situation the skin incision may be enlarged to allow good visualisation of the muscular layers. Airtightness of this port depends on a small opening in the muscles which is snug around the port, and not on a small skin incision. This is less of a concern if using ports with a self-retaining balloon.

A large first port with gas leak: Leakage from a loose first port can lead to surgical emphysema and gas loss. This problem can be solved by inserting a piece of plain or alternatively petroleum jelly-impregnated gauze beside the port and tying the stay sutures tight, thus preventing leak.

Anatomy obscured by plentiful retroperitoneal fat: Temporary elevation of gas pressure may improve visibility. An attempt should be made to ascertain whether the fat is paranephric (outside Gerota's fascia) or perinephric (inside Gerota's fascia). Paranephric fat may be excised taking care not to injure the peritoneum. Excision of paranephric fat must be done with Harmonic Scalpel or LigaSure to avoid bleeding. Following excision of paranephric fat placing it in the lower part of the space, the Gerota's fascia is visualised and can be opened close to the psoas muscle.

Minor bleeders in the renal hilum: A pledget of gauze applied for a few minutes is usually efficacious in causing haemostasis.

Peritoneal rent causing loss of pneumoretroperitoneum: A Veress needle is placed in the peritoneal cavity to reduce intraperitoneal pressure. If this is ineffective, the tear may be closed by applying a row of 5 mm clips to approximate the edges.

RLDN in special situations: RLDN is effective in donors with multiple renal arteries [15] (Fig. 8.10). It has also been used in cases with precaval renal arteries on the right side [16], multiple right renal veins [17] and IVC duplication with short left renal veins [18]. Excellent exposure of renal vasculature facilitates management of anomalous vessels.

8.4 Discussion

Laparoscopic donor nephrectomy is now widely used and has the advantages of reducing donor morbidity, shortening time to return of normal activities [19] and reducing disincentives to living kidney donation [20]. However safety concerns persist, and adverse events occur and are probably under-reported [21]. LDN converts what was traditionally an extraperitoneal operation into a transperitoneal one, with potential for bowel-related complications. Thus a technique which combines the advantages of a minimal access approach with the advantages of an extraperitoneal operation would seem to be advantageous. RLDN offers rapid exposure of the Gerota's fascia and its contents. The renal hilum is directly visualised, and the distance between the ports and the vessels is less, allowing more precise movements and better visualisation.

In RLDN intraperitoneal viscera such as the small bowel, liver and spleen are kept out of the operative field and less likely to be injured. In addition postoperative ileus may be less than in LDN as bowel is not manipulated. The major cause of readmission after living donor nephrectomy is bowel related, including ileus, vomiting and abdominal distension [22].

A number of large series of RLDN attest to its safety and efficacy. Yoshimura et al. [23] compared RLDN with open donor nephrectomy ODN. They found similar warm ischaemia times, longer operative time and shorter hospitalisation time for RLDN. There were no instances of delayed graft function in patients who underwent RLDN. Similarly Bachmann et al. found no statistically significant differences in recipient outcome, operative time and cold ischaemia time in a retrospective non-randomised comparison of RLDN and ODN [24]. Tanabe et al. reported their experience with 135 consecutive donors who underwent RLDN [25]. In this series return of bowel function took 0.7 days, 4.9 days to discharge and 12 days to return to work. There was one conversion and no major complications and all grafts showed primary function. Kohei et al. reviewed 425 RLDNs performed at a single centre [26]. All recipients achieved normal serum creatinine levels, and 1-year graft survival was 98.2%. RLND is associated with significantly reduced postoperative pain compared to ODN [27]. Ruszat et al. compared RLDN with ODN, LDN and hand-assisted LDN [28]. They reported that RLDN had significantly shorter operative times compared to LDN and HLDN. Warm ischaemia time was shorter with ODN and RLDN compared to LDN. RLDN had less blood loss and shorter hospitalisation that LDN in their series.

Bachmann et al. compared early complications of RLDN with ODN and found no significant difference in major and minor complications in the two groups [24]. Tanabe et al. in a series of 135 cases encountered no major complications and six minor complications including pulmonary embolism which was managed conservatively and transfusion requirement in one patient [25]. Similarly Ruszat et al. found no significant differences in complication rates when they compared ODN, LDN, RLDN and hand-assisted RLDN [28]. Ma et al. reported no blood transfusion or conversion in a series of 138 patients and found a decline in complication rates from 22.5 to 7.5% from the first 40 donors to the second 40 donors, suggesting the learning curve for RLDN [29]. Kohei et al. reported one conversion and an overall complication rate of 4.9%. One donor had a nonfatal pulmonary embolism and no donor required readmission [26]. No mortality was reported in any of these series.

Obesity is not a contraindication to RLDN, and indeed RLDN has certain advantages in this population of donors. While in the flank position, the pannus of fat falls towards the contralateral side and away from the flank. This is of advantage in obese donors, in whom abundant fat can obscure landmarks and make port placement difficult. In contrast, in LDN, the fat pannus falls towards the site of port placement.

RLDN can be safely used in right donor nephrectomy [30, 31]. Control of the right renal vein is problematic, and some published series of LDN have low numbers of right-sided kidneys [32]. RLDN allows the stapler to be deployed parallel to the IVC, thus making it possible to place the staples on the IVC and avoiding loss of renal vein length, and taking a cuff of the IVC, which makes suturing easier during the recipient operation [14]. Retro-caval dissection of the right renal vein is facilitated, and the dissection can be carried till the origin of the right renal artery on the aorta if necessary. This is of benefit in cases with early branching of the right renal artery where it is desirous to get a common stump, which would necessitate an inter-aortocaval dissection in LDN.

Being an extraperitoneal operation, in RLDN postoperative collections are confined to the retroperitoneum. Chyloperitoneum following laparoscopic donor nephrectomy is attended by considerable morbidity and can require reoperation for its management [33]. Chyloretroperitoneum following RLDN is more likely to be amenable to nonoperative management [34]. In the event of catastrophic postoperative loss of vascular control, bleeding would be limited to the retroperitoneal space, and a tamponade effect would limit the extent of blood loss.

Port-site hernia is unlikely following RLDN as the intact peritoneum and retroperitoneal fat prevent herniation of intra-abdominal viscera.

Pneumoperitoneum has been shown to reduce renal blood flow and may contribute to ischaemia of the renal graft [35]. Chiu et al. reported that the effect of unilateral pneumoretroperitoneum is less than of pneumoperitoneum [36]. It is critical to keep gas pressures as low as possible to optimise graft function.

RLND does not require any special instruments that are not available in any surgical set-up that routinely performs laparoscopy. The balloon is indigenously made and low cost, and no special disposables are required. This is of importance in developing countries, where cost considerations are critical [37].

RLND is still not as widely practised as LDN. Reasons for this include unfamiliarity with retroperitoneal anatomy and unfamiliarity with laparoscopy among surgeons without a urological background, as well as concerns about graft function and donor safety. At our institute we have performed over 2,500 RLDNs since 2003. Retroperitoneal laparoscopy should be easily adopted by urologists as they are familiar with retroperitoneal anatomy. We perform retroperitoneal laparoscopy regularly for indications such as ablative nephrectomy, radical nephrectomy, partial nephrectomy, adrenalectomy and ureterolithotomy. Our trainees and junior consultants follow a graded introduction or RLDN, where they perform non-donor retroperitoneal laparoscopy, assist an experienced surgeon in RLDN and perform the operation under supervision and then independently. A number of our trainees are now practising RLND at other centres in India. We believe that RLDN is a safe operation that results in good donor and recipient outcomes. It can be taught and replicated and is a technique that deserves to be popularised among the transplant community.

References

1. Cecka JM. Clinical transplants 1995. In: Cecka JM, PI T, editors. Living donor transplants. Los Angeles: UCLA Tissue Typing Laboratory; 1995. p. 363.
2. Chatterjee S, Nam R, Fleshner N, Klotz L. Permanent flank bulge is a consequence of flank incision for radical nephrectomy in one half of patients. Urol Oncol. 2004;22:36.
3. Yang SC, Rha KH, Kim YS, et al. Retroperitoneoscopic-assisted living donor nephrectomy: 109 cases. Transplant Proc. 2001;33:1104.
4. Ratner LE, Ciseck LJ, Moore RG, et al. Laparoscopic live donor nephrectomy. Transplantation. 1995;60:1047.
5. Wadstrom J. Hand-assisted retroperitoneoscopic live donor nephrectomy: experience from the first 75 consecutive cases. Transplantation. 2005;80(8):1060.
6. Gershbein AB, Fuchs. Hand assisted and conventional live donor nephrectomy: a; comparison of two contemporary techniques. J Endourol. 2002;16(7):509–13.
7. Lindstrom P, Haggman M, Wadstrom J. Hand assisted laparoscopic surgery (HALS) is more time and cost-effective than standard laparoscopic nephrectomy. Surg Endosc. 2002;16(3):422.

8. Greenstein MA, Harkaway R, Bodosa, et al. Minimal incision open living nephrectomy compared to hand assisted laparoscopic living donor nephrectomy. World J Urol. 2003;20:356.
9. Gaur DD. Laparoscopic operative retroperitoneoscopy: use of a new device. J Urol. 1992;148(4):1137–9.
10. Gill IS, Uzzo RG, Hobart MG, et al. Laparoscopic retroperitoneal live donor right nephrectomy for purposes of allotransplantation and autotransplantation. J Urol. 2000;164:1500.
11. A report of the Amsterdam forum on the care of the live kidney donor: data and medical guidelines. Transplantation 2005; 79: S53–S66.
12. Modi PR, Goel R, Dodia S. Retroperitoneoscopic left donor nephrectomy: use of Hem-o-lok clips for control of renal pedicle. J Endourol. 2007;21:1029–31.
13. Simforoosh N, Aminsharifi A, Zand S, et al. How to improve the safety of polymer clips during laparoscopic donor nephrectomy. J Endourol. 2007;21:1319–22.
14. Modi P, Kadam G, Devra A. Obtaining a cuff of inferior vena cava by use of the endo-TA stapler in retroperitoneoscopic right-side donor nephrectomy. Urology. 2007;69(5):832.
15. Omoto K, Nozaki T, Inui M, et al. Retroperitoneoscopic donor nephrectomy with multiple renal arteries does not affect graft survival and ureteral complications. Transplantation. 2014;98:1175.
16. Modi PR, Rizvi SJ, Gupta R. Retroperitoneoscopic right-sided donor nephrectomy with pre- and postcaval renal arteries. Urology. 2008;72:672.
17. Modi PR, Rizvi SJ. Two renal veins are not a contraindication to retroperitoneoscopic right donor nephrectomy. J Endourol. 2008;22(7):1491.
18. Rizvi SJ, Prasad TK, Modi PR. Retroperitoneoscopic left donor nephrectomy with duplicated IVC. Indian J Nephrol. 2012;22(6):480–1.
19. Velidedeoglu E, Williams N, Brayman KL, et al. Comparison of open, laparoscopic and hand assisted approaches to live-donor nephrectomy. Transplantation. 2002;74:169–72.
20. Schweitzer EJ, Wilson J, Jacobs S, et al. Increased rates of donation with laparoscopic donor nephrectomy. Ann Surg. 2000;232:392.
21. Shokeir AA. Open versus laparoscopic live donor nephrectomy: a focus on the safety of donors and the need for a donor registry. J Urol. 2007;178(5):1860–6.
22. Chin EH, Hazzan D, Edye M, et al. The first decade of a laparoscopic donor nephrectomy program: effect of surgeon and institution experience with 512 cases from 1996 to 2006. J Am Coll Surg. 2009;209:106.
23. Yoshimura K, Takahara S, Kyakuno M, et al. J Endourol. 2005;19(7):808.
24. Bachmann A, Wolff T, Ruszat R, et al. Retroperitoneoscopic donor nephrectomy: a retrospective, non-randomised comparison of early complications, donor and recipient outcome with the standard open approach. Eur Urol. 2005;48:90–6.
25. Tanabe K, Miyamoto N, Ishida H. Retroperitoneoscopic live donor nephrectomy (RPLDN): Establishment and initial experience of RPLDN at a single centre. Am J Transplant. 2005;5:739.
26. Kohei N, Kazuya O, Hirai T, et al. Retroperitoneoscopic living donor nephrectomy: experience of 425 cases at a single centre. J Endourol. 2010;24(11):1783.
27. Bachmann A, Wolff T, Giannini O, et al. How painful is donor nephrectomy? Retrospective analysis of early pain and pain management in open versus laparoscopic versus retroperitoneoscopic nephrectomy. Transplantation. 2006;81(12):1735.
28. Ruszat R, Sulser T, Dickenmann M, et al. Retroperitoneoscopic donor nephrectomy: donor outcome and complication rate in comparison with three different techniques. World J Urol. 2006;24:113.
29. Ma L, Ye J, Huang Y, et al. Retroperitoneoscopic live-donor nephrectomy: 5-year single-centre experience in China. Int J Urol. 2010;17:158.
30. Ruszat R, Wyler SF, Wolff T, et al. Reluctance over right-sided retroperitoneoscopic living donor nephrectomy: justified or not? Transplant Proc. 2007;39:1381–5.
31. Gao Z, Wu J, Yang D. Retroperitoneoscopic right living donor nephrectomy. Chin Med J. 2007;120(14):1270.

32. Jacobs S, Cho E, Foster C, et al. Laparoscopic donor nephrectomy: the University of Maryland 6-year experience. J Urol. 2004;171:47–51.
33. Aerts J, Matas A, Sutherland D, et al. Chylous ascites requiring surgical intervention after donor nephrectomy: case series and single centre experience. Am J Transplant. 2010;10(1):124.
34. Sharma S, Rizvi SJ, Modi PR. Medical management of chyloretroperitoneum following retroperitoneoscopic donor nephrectomy. Indian J Nephrol. 2014;24(2):139.
35. Burgos FJ, Pascual J, Briones G, et al. Influence of laparoscopic live donor nephrectomy in ischemia-reperfusion syndrome and renal function after kidney transplantation: and experimental study. Transplant Proc. 2003;35:1664–5.
36. Chiu AW, Chang LS, Burkitt DH. The impact of pneumoperitoneum, pneumoretroperitoneum and gasless laparoscopy on the systemic and renal hemodynamics. J Am Coll Surg. 1995;181(5):397.
37. Ye J, Huang Y, Hou X. Retroperitoneal laparoscopic live donor nephrectomy: a cost-effective approach. Urology. 2010;75(1):92–5.

Laparoendoscopic Single-Site Surgery Donor Nephrectomy (LESS DN)

Pradeep Rao and Abraham Kurien

Abstract

Laparoscopic donor nephrectomy is now the gold standard in retrieving grafts from living donors. LESS DN is not much different from the standard laparoscopic technique. The surgical view and steps of both surgeries are the same. The main difference would be the singular skin incision and its consequence. The consequence to the patient is lesser pain, faster return to normal activity, and improved cosmesis. The consequence to the surgeon is the challenge of the learning curve. If eating with hands and eating with fork and spoon were open donor nephrectomy and laparoscopic donor nephrectomy, respectively, then eating with chopsticks is LESS DN! The learning curve is in understanding and overcoming the restriction in hand movements. The chapter takes the reader through the challenges and technique of LESS DN.

9.1 What Is LESS DN?

Laparoendoscopic single-site surgery donor nephrectomy (LESS DN) is a result of natural development of minimally invasive surgery to further decrease morbidity to the donor and a move in the direction toward a scarless surgery. Standard laparoscopic donor nephrectomy (LDN) was first reported in 1995 [1]. It was an attempt to reduce the morbidity for a group of people undergoing surgery for purely altruistic

P. Rao (✉)
Global Hospitals, Mumbai, Maharashtra, India
e-mail: pprao@mac.com

A. Kurien
Madras Medical Mission, Chennai, Tamil Nadu, India
e-mail: abrkurien@gmail.com

© Springer Nature Singapore Pte Ltd. 2017
M.R. Desai, A.P. Ganpule (eds.), *Laparoscopic Donor Nephrectomy*,
DOI 10.1007/978-981-10-2849-6_9

reasons. Over the next few years, LDN increased the donor pool and became accepted as the gold standard for donor nephrectomy [2–4]. In LESS DN, donor nephrectomy is performed through ports deployed through a single small incision with extraction of the graft also through the same incision. As with most other LESS procedures, the aim is to improve cosmesis as well as reduce pain for the donor.

9.2 Terminology

The first report of single-port nephrectomy was in 2007 [5]. Since then, most ablative and reconstructive urologic surgeries have been performed using this technique.

Various terminologies were applied for this method of single-site surgery including single-port access (SPA), one-port umbilical surgery (OPUS), natural orifice transumbilical surgery (NOTUS), transumbilical endoscopic surgery (TUES), transumbilical laparoscopic-assisted (TULA) surgery, and embryonic natural orifice transluminal endoscopic surgery (ENOTES). To determine a universally acceptable name for single-incision laparoscopic surgery, a multidisciplinary consortium of experts, the Laparoendoscopic Single-Site Surgery Consortium for Assessment and Research (LESSCAR), met in 2008. The consortium determined that "laparoendoscopic single-site surgery (LESS)" was both scientifically accurate and colloquially appropriate, and, therefore, the term was ratified by the NOTES Working Group of the Endourological Society and was adapted as the future standard for the reference [6].

There were two distinct techniques of access used under this umbrella of LESS, by using various access devices which permitted multiple instruments or by using three to four separate trocars through a single site, either umbilical or through a Pfannenstiel incision. Both these approaches have been used for LESS DN [7, 8].

9.3 Problems with LESS Donor Nephrectomy

The technique of LESS donor nephrectomy is more challenging as compared to LDN. Studies comparing LESS DN versus LDN have noted that LESS DN is more challenging [9, 10]. Any new technique is never without challenges. Understanding these challenges is very important in overcoming them.

9.3.1 Extracorporeal Challenges

9.3.1.1 Clashing of Surgeon's Own Hands

Laparoscopic surgery is counterintuitive. Working ports are placed next to each other and are usually aligned craniocaudally, with the patient in a lateral position. To move the intracorporeal working end of the instrument cranially, the hand holding the instrument extracorporeally is moved in the caudal direction and vice versa (Fig. 9.1).

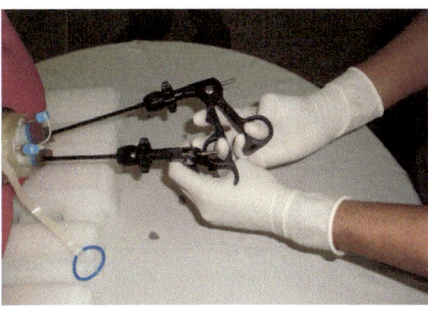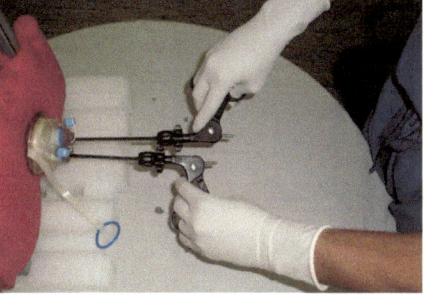

Fig. 9.1 Clashing of instruments and hands. Learn to hold instruments in a different manner so to avoid clashing of hands

In LESS DN, since both hands are held close to each other, in a craniocaudal working port arrangement, the caudal hand restricts the caudal moment of the cranial hand. Similarly, the cranial hand restricts the cranial movement of the caudal hand. There is no restriction to either hand to move medially or laterally with ports in the craniocaudal axis. Similarly, if the working ports are arranged in a medial-lateral axis, the lateral hand will restrict the lateral movement of the medial hand, and similarly the medial hand will restrict the medial movement of the lateral hand. There is no restriction to either hand to move cranially and caudally with ports in the medial-lateral axis. Understanding this extracorporeal restriction of hand movement is crucial in modifying your hand movements in LESS.

9.3.1.2 Clashing of Surgeon's Hands with Cameraman's Hands
Clashing of the surgeon's hands with the cameraman's hands is a possibility in LESS DN due to the close proximity of the camera port to the working ports. So, depending upon the location of the cameraman's hand, the movement of the surgeon's hands in that direction would be restricted.

9.3.1.3 Damage to Accessory Equipment
In LESS DN, the window of entry to the abdomen is narrow. Apart from surgeon's and assistant's hands, the limited extracorporeal space is packed with the instruments and accessories including various cables, cords, and tubings. If not careful, some of these accessories like the light cable can easily get damaged between clashing working instruments. We have found video laparoscopes which have in-line light cables causing the least amount of clashing with the instruments.

9.3.2 Intracorporeal Challenges

9.3.2.1 Lack of Triangulation
Triangulation is one of the fundamental concepts of laparoscopic surgery, as it permits traction and counter traction on tissues to facilitate dissection along anatomical planes. A comfortable triangulation, with two ports kept many centimeters apart like

in LDN, is not achieved with LESS DN. When you are dissecting head-on with hands held close to each other, the angle of triangulation is very acute. When the hands holding the instruments are not held close to each other, the instruments tend to cross each other. The instrument held by the right hand crosses over to the left and vice versa.

9.3.2.2 Lack of Assistant Retraction Ports

In LDN, the uretero-gonadal packet can be retracted away by an assistant with an instrument inserted through a lateral port, achieving gentle traction while dissecting the pedicle. Similarly, instruments can help in retracting other organs like the bowel, spleen, and liver to improve your vision on the area of dissection as and when required by placing appropriate extra ports. These assistant retraction ports can be placed in LESS DN but will further contribute to the clashing of hands and instruments.

9.3.3   Solutions to the Problems

9.3.3.1 Switching of Ports

The extracorporeal clashing of surgeon's hands to a certain extent can be avoided by switching the instrument ports. The caudal hand instrument is shifted into the cranial port, and the cranial hand instrument is shifted to the caudal port. So the dominant instrument held by the right hand (by a right handed surgeon) is now held by the left hand. The retraction instrument is held by the right hand. The surgeon should develop skills to do few surgical steps with the nondominant hand. If the surgeon is uncomfortable in operating the dominant instrument with the left hand, he may cross the hands extracorporeally. By crossing hands, the dominant working instrument can continue to be operated by the dominant hand. Another option which is possible in some access device is to switch the orientation of the working ports from a craniocaudal arrangement to a medial-lateral configuration (Fig. 9.2).

9.3.3.2 Use Instruments of Differing Lengths

Another way to prevent clashing of hands is to use instruments of different lengths. So one instrument can be of standard length, while the other instrument is of bariatric length. The hands will then be kept away from each other extracorporeally, by keeping them in different planes of movement (Fig. 9.3).

9.3.3.3 Cameraman Sits Down

The cameraman should sit down to maximize the extracorporeal work space for the surgeon who is standing. It also helps if the cameraman holds the camera by its "tail," rather than by the regular grip, so as to give more space to the surgeon (Fig. 9.4).

9.3.3.4 Use of Thinner Laparoscope

The clashing of working instruments with the laparoscope can occur frequently (Fig. 9.5). The clashing of instruments can be avoided by using thinner 5 mm laparoscopes instead of the standard 10 mm laparoscope.

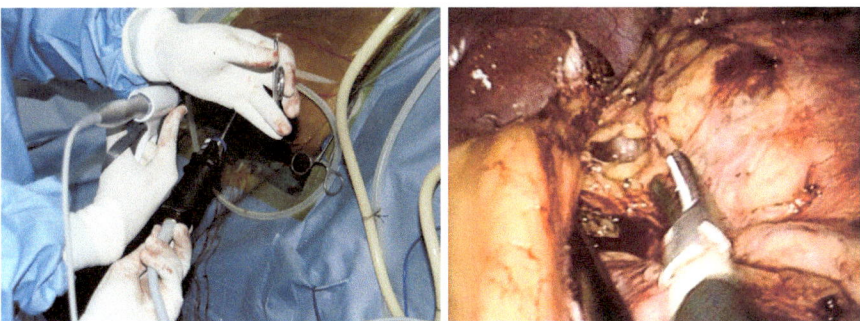

Fig. 9.2 The upper pole dissection is facilitated by switching ports

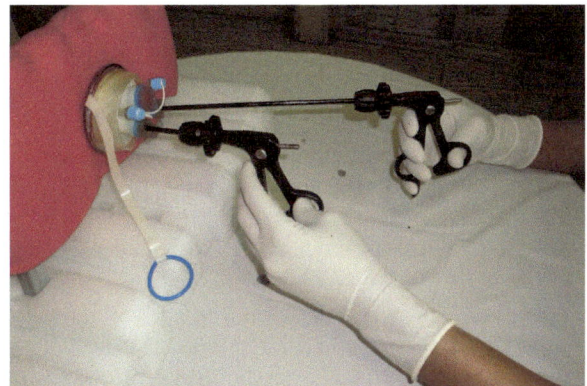

Fig. 9.3 Longer working instruments help to keep away the working hand from the retracting hand

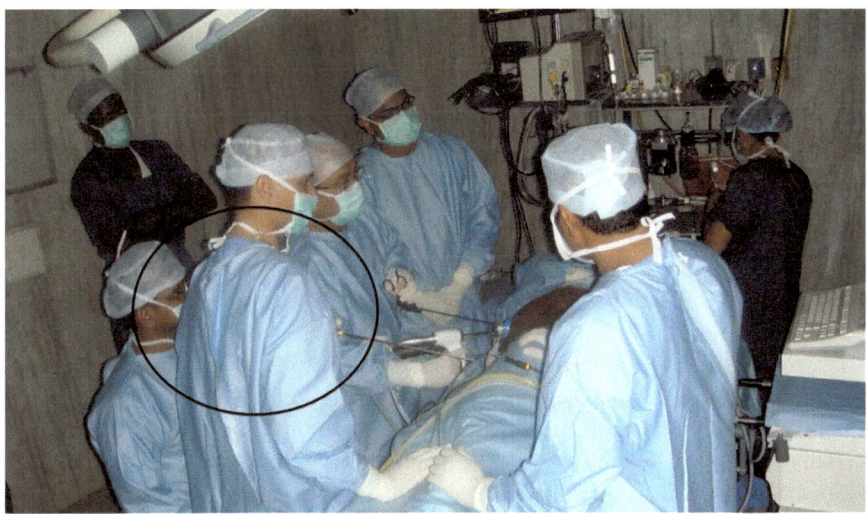

Fig. 9.4 To improve the ergonomics, the camera driver sits and surgeon stands

Fig. 9.5 Nutcracker effect, the light pillar of a conventional telescope causes clashing with the retracting and working instruments

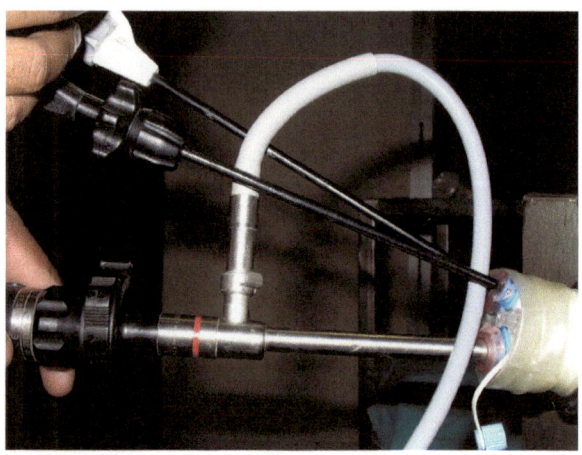

9.3.3.5 Use of Longer Laparoscope

A longer bariatric laparoscope will keep the cameraman's hand holding the camera further away from the surgeon, thus giving the surgeon more space.

9.3.3.6 Use of Laparoscope with Coaxial Light and Optic Cable

The regular light cable with its perpendicular entry into the laparoscope from the top invariably gets onto the way of the surgeon's working instruments. Sometimes, these light cables may also get crushed and damaged. The Endo Eye (Olympus, Tokyo, Japan) was suited for this as it came with the "chip-on-tip" technology which meant that it has a streamlined profile with a single coaxial cable and this reduced the cluttering and clashing with the bulky camera head and light cable.

9.3.3.7 Cameraman's Hands Kept Away Down Under

In LDN, the laparoscope is placed at a slightly lower plane of view as compared to the working instruments. In LESS DN, the laparoscope is best placed in such a way as to get a bird's-eye view of the working instruments. The advantage being, the hand holding the laparoscope, is kept away below the surgeon's hands. A deflectable tip 5 mm laparoscope with a coaxial light cable is ideal for performing LESS procedures [5]. But a deflectable tip laparoscope would require the cameraman to be well versed and knowledgeable in its movements (Fig. 9.6).

9.3.3.8 Use of Articulating Instrumentation

Articulating instrumentation allows for triangulation or at least the effect to occur intracorporeally despite the entry points being adjacent to one another through the same skin incision. Articulating instruments were originally developed to mimic the freedom of movement afforded by the robotic wrist of the da Vinci Surgical Robot (Intuitive Surgical, Sunnyvale, CA). Articulating graspers, Endo Shears (Autosuture, Norwalk, CT), and needle holders are available. Roticulating instruments (Covidien, Dublin, Ireland) have a 0–80° range of motion, allowing infinite freedom for tip

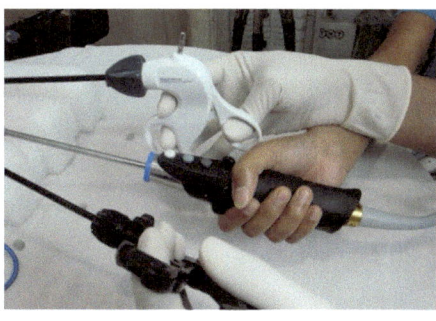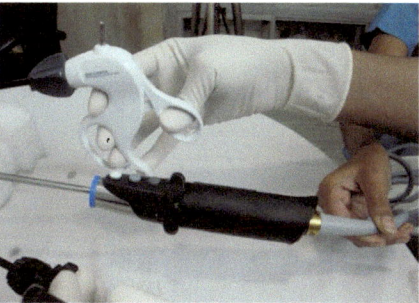

Fig. 9.6 Holding the camera as distal as possible also keeps the cameraman's hands away from the surgeon's hands. This prevents what is called as clashing swords

adjustment. They have a spin lock mechanism that allows them to use it as a rigid instrument. Handheld Autonomy Laparo-Angle Instruments (Cambridge Endo, Framingham, MA) have been designed to simulate the surgeons hand in motion and, with its axial rotation knob and exclusive angle locking mechanism, provide a better control. One disadvantage is that using all these articulating instruments has a significant learning curve before one handles them dexterously. The major disadvantage with most of the available articulating instruments is a lack of strength to retract using these. The cutting instruments like the hook or the scissors are most useful among the articulating instruments. Another issue is that by necessity, ultrasonic shears can neither be bent nor articulating.

9.3.3.9 Use of Prebent Instruments

Prebent instruments also attempt to achieve triangulation intracorporeally and also attempt to keep the hands away extracorporeally. Prebent instruments cannot be passed through regular straight trocars. They can, however, be passed through some of the access devices like the GelPOINT™, TriPort™, and QuadPort™, which have a very low profile inside and outside the abdominal wall. The advantage of the prebent instruments is that they have a fair degree of strength and can be used for retraction.

Our present recommendation for LESS is to use a prebent instrument for retraction in the left hand and a straight instrument for dissection and cutting in the right hand (Fig. 9.7).

9.3.3.10 Use of Deflectable Tip Laparoscope

A 5 mm laparoscope with a flexible, actively deflectable tip can be used. If a deflectable tip laparoscope is used, the cameraman's hands can be positioned in a dependent position, away from the surgeon's hands, and the tip deflected downward for a bird's-eye view of the surgical field. The tip can be bent up to 100 ° in four directions. This means that relevant area can be thoroughly examined head-on, from above and from behind. Once bend the tip can be locked in that position to decrease the fatigue of the operator (Fig. 9.8).

Fig. 9.7 The prebent
instrument in one hand
helps in decreasing
intracorporeal clashing

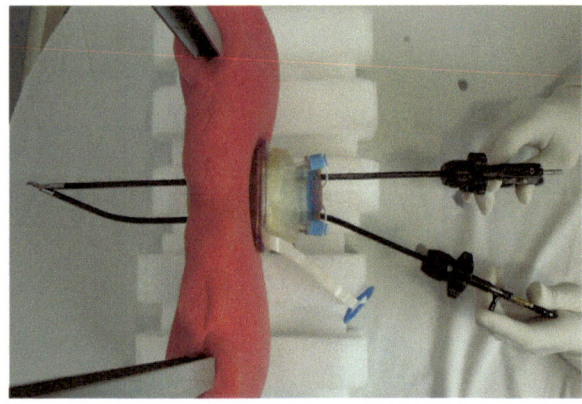

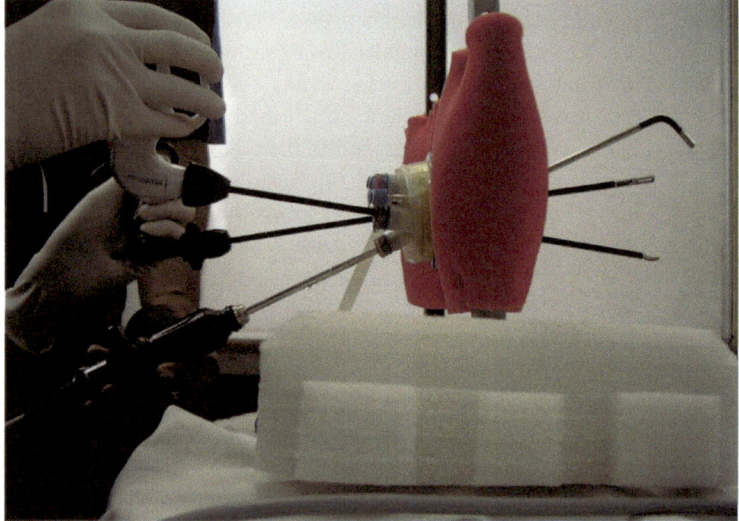

Fig. 9.8 A flexible tip telescope does a remarkable job at staying in a vantage point with a good
view and staying away from the surgeon's movement

9.3.3.11 Technique of Disentangling Laparoscope

When the instruments get entangled with the laparoscope, the maneuver to separate
is to pull back the laparoscope (without coming out of the port) till it disentangles
and then push the laparoscope forward with a slight upward tilt. The purpose is to
keep the laparoscope above and look down onto the working instruments so as to
keep the cameraman's hands down and away from surgeon's hands (Fig. 9.9).

9.3.3.12 Use of an Additional Retraction Instrument

A pediatric 3 mm port with a 3 mm long grasper can be used to give traction if
required to assist in specific steps of the surgery, at least till the learning curve of the
surgeon is overcome. A fascial (port) closure needle (Karl Storz GmBH and co,

Fig. 9.9 Positioning the telescope at a vantage point helps in optimal dissection

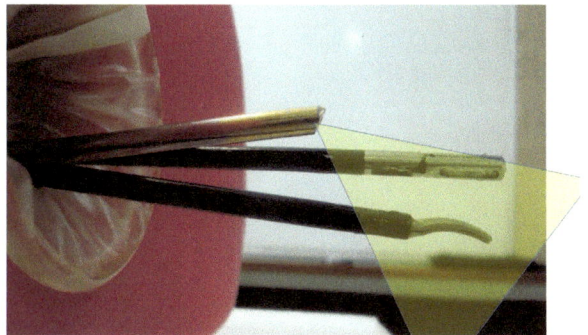

Tuttlingen, Germany) can also be used for retraction without the need of a port. It is directly punctured and inserted intra-abdominally through the subcostal region. The upper part of an infant feeding tube is cut and fed into an open end of a plastic needle cap. The cap is inserted into the abdomen through one of the 10 mm ports. The port closure needle is passed into the open end of the needle cap through the rubber of the feeding tube. This arrangement allows for a snug and secure placement of the port closure needle into the needle cap. This assembly is used to provide traction to the kidney and adjacent organs [11].

9.4 Access Devices for LESS DN

LESS DN has been performed through an umbilical or Pfannenstiel incision [7, 8]. Standard ports can be inserted through the same skin incision by using separate fascial punctures. There are also various access devices available that can be deployed through the single incision to facilitate easy insertion of multiple instruments. Some of these access devices are reusable.

There have been a variety of access devices used for LESS. Most of them are now off the market or unavailable. The two devices which seem to have endured are the Olympus QuadPort Plus and the Applied medical GelPOINT device. In addition, LESS is carried out using shorter trocars put in through a single incision.

The Olympus QuadPort is a disposable, multi-instrument access device designed to facilitate laparoendoscopic single-site (LESS) surgery. The QuadPort contains five instrument ports and two valves. One valve is for insufflation and the other one for smoke evacuation. There are five instrument ports (two 5 mm, one 10 mm, one 12 mm, and one 15 mm). These flexible ports accommodate different types and sizes of laparoscopic instruments, including straight, curved, and articulating instruments. Duckbill/lipseal valves allow for easy introduction and removal of instruments while maintaining pneumoperitoneum. A removal ribbon enables easy device removal (Fig. 9.10). The GelPOINT device is similar and can be used with or without trocars through the gel valve.

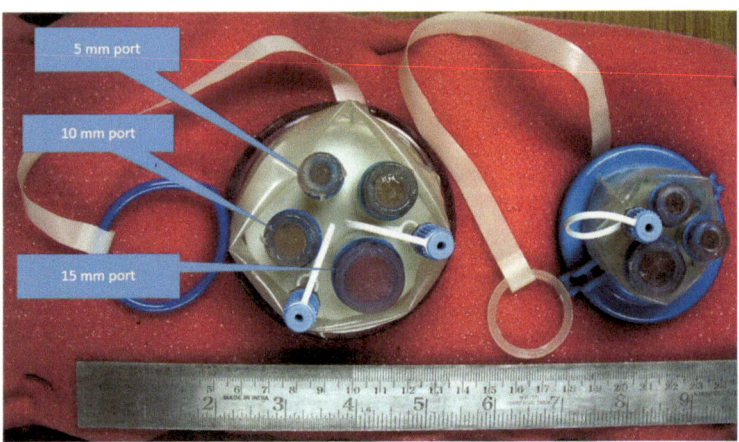

Fig. 9.10 The variants of TriPort and QuadPort

X-Cone (Karl Storz – Endoskope, Tuttlingen, Germany), with five openings 10/12 mm and 5 mm×4, is reusable access device but has not been reported for use in LESS DN.

9.4.1 Our Technique

The patient once under general anesthesia is positioned in lateral position after placing a nasogastric tube or orogastric tube for decompressing the stomach. A Foley's urethral catheter is routinely placed to monitor urine output. All pressure points are well padded. The patient is also adequately strapped to the table. After cleaning and draping the patient. An umbilical incision of approximately 4.5 cm length is made and deepened to the sheath. The sheath and peritoneum are incised to 5.5 cm. An Olympus QuadPort+ is deployed using the introducer.

We mostly use a 5 mm, 30° Olympus laparoscope with integrated camera head and coaxial light cable (Endoeye HD II 5 mm). Regular rigid instruments are usually used even though curved and articulating instruments are available. Ten millimeter instruments like the Hem-o-lok applicator, 12 mm instruments like Endo GIA or Endo TA laparoscopic staplers, and 15 mm Endo Catch II specimen retrieval pouch can easily be inserted through the 12 or 15 mm ports. Lubricating the shaft of the instruments with water helps in decreasing the friction and easy movement in and through the ports.

The steps of LESS DN are identical to LDN.

9.4.1.1 Colonic Reflection

The colon is reflected after incising the white line of Toldt. Care is taken not to disturb the kidney with its Gerota's fascia while dropping the colon. The splenorenal ligament is incised so as to drop the spleen medially. This also helps in dropping the splenic flexure.

9.4.1.2 Uretero-gonadal Packet Mobilization

The gonadal vein and the ureter are identified and they are lifted off the psoas muscle along with the surrounding fat enclosed within the Gerota's fascia. Once this packet is lifted out, the renal vein comes into view.

9.4.1.3 Adrenal Vein Division

Once the renal vein comes into view, the adrenal vein is identified. While mobilizing, the adrenal vein care must be taken to watch out for an inferior phrenic vein which sometimes drains into the adrenal vein. The adrenal vein is clipped with Hem-o-lok clips and divided.

9.4.2 Upper Pole Separation

Soon after dividing the adrenal vein the upper pole along with the adrenal gland is lifted off the psoas. The Gerota's fascia is incised to expose the upper pole. The adrenal gland is separated off the upper pole of kidney using ultrasonic shears as this tissue contains small adrenal arteries branching from the renal artery. Switching of ports may be required during upper pole dissection. Bariatric extra-long instruments are useful in dissecting the upper pole of kidney especially an extra-long ultrasonic shear.

9.4.3 Lumbar Vein Division

The aorta just inferior to left renal vein crossing is exposed. The periaortic fat tissue is divided to expose the renal artery. Usually at this level, we come across the lumbar veins which are meticulously dissected out and divided between Hem-o-lok clips. Occasionally, we do not come across a lumbar vein draining into the renal vein.

9.4.4 Renal Pedicle Dissection

Once the lumbar vein is divided, the renal artery comes well into our view. All the loose fatty tissue containing neural and lymphatic tissue surrounding the renal artery and vein are divided for complete mobilization of the renal vessels.

9.4.5 Division of the Gonadal Vein and Ureter

Once the recipient surgeon is ready to receive the graft, the ureter and gonadal vein are clipped and divided at the level of the pelvic brim. The lateral attachment to the kidney is divided up to the upper pole. A small strip of lateral attachment is left at the mid pole so that the kidney does not drop medially.

9.4.6   Division of the Renal Pedicle

The kidney is lifted off the aorta so as to straighten the renal vessels with a retracting instrument. The renal artery is then doubly clipped with Hem-o-lok clips and divided so that a 2 mm cuff remains with the clips. The vein is then doubly clipped and divided.

9.4.7   Graft Retrieval

The small strip of lateral attachment is incised with cold scissors. The Gerota's fascia of the freed graft is held with a laparoscopic grasper and the graft gently moved toward the QuadPort. The removal ribbon is pulled which dislodge the QuadPort. Using a thick open-surgery scissors, the sheath may be further incised, extending the sheath incision by 1–2 cm. The skin incision rarely needs to be extended. The technique of graft retrieval in LESS DN is different from LDN. In LDN, through the retrieval incision, the surgeon's hand can be introduced with ease to retrieve the graft. In LESS DN, since the single-port incision is smaller, the surgeon's hand cannot be inserted to retrieve the graft. But the surgeon's fingers (index finger, middle finger, and thumb) can go across the incised opening, to hold and gently remove the graft which was brought toward the exit by the laparoscopic grasper.

An Endo Catch II specimen retrieval pouch introduced through the 15 mm port can also be used to retrieve the graft. Another technique helping in graft retrieval is to pull the graft toward the incision along its transverse axis by a no. 1 Vicryl suture tied laparoscopically around the fat along with the gonadal vein [11]. This suture is tied and exteriorized, prior to division of renal pedicle, through one of the ports. Once the renal vessels are clipped and divided, the suture is gently pulled, and the graft aligned vertically is gently retrieved through the incision.

9.5 Scientific Evidence

There are a few randomized trials comparing LDN with LESS DN. Kurien et al. [9] in a randomized controlled trial (RCT) comparing outcomes in 25 cases of LESS DN to 25 cases of LDN revealed that there was early relief of pain and shorter hospital stay in patients who underwent LESS DN. The warm ischemia time (WIT) was longer in LESS DN even though the early graft function was similar in both groups. The blood loss, intraoperative, and postoperative complications were comparable in both groups. This study used an umbilical incision with a QuadPort device and retrieval of the graft seemed to be difficult. Richstone et al. [8] used a Pfannenstiel incision and randomized patients for 2 years. With a total of 29 patients, they found significantly less pain with LESS donors. Autorino et al. [10] in a systematic review and meta-analysis of nine studies (two RCTs and seven retrospective studies) comparing LESS DN and LDN, involving 461 LESS DN cases and 1,006 LDN cases, concluded that LESS DN offers comparable surgical and early functional outcomes to conventional LDN, with a lower analgesic requirement. LESS DN represents an emerging option for living kidney donation.

9.6   Why LESS DN?

A live kidney donor is not a patient with a disease that needs cure. The donor is an altruistic person with an intention to save the life of the recipient. This donation is truly a selfless gift of life. Even then, there are many disincentives for a person to donate for their loved ones. These include the morbidity of the surgery including pain and delayed return to normal activities. The donor deserves to have the least morbidity and an earlier return to normal daily activities.

Multiple-port standard laparoscopic donor nephrectomy became the gold standard in many institutions as it offered the donors reduced postoperative pain, faster recovery, and better cosmesis over open donor nephrectomy. In LDN, the precise dissection achieved due to excellent imaging and wide space created with pneumoperitoneum results in fewer complications and decreased blood loss. The reduced morbidity of LDN has augmented the number of live donors coming forward to donate for their loved ones [12]. LESS DN has evolved with an aim not only to decrease the number of incisions and associated better cosmesis but also to further reduce postoperative pain, reduce wound-related complications, and quicker convalescence. LESS DN has the potential to further decrease the barriers and disincentives to kidney donation.

References

1. Ratner LE, Ciseck LJ, Moore RG, Cigarroa FG, Kaufman HS, Kavoussi LR. Laparoscopic live donor nephrectomy. Transplantation. 1995;60(9):1047–9.
2. Ratner LE, Kavoussi LR, Sroka M, Hiller J, Weber R, Schulam PG, et al. Laparoscopic assisted live donor nephrectomy – a comparison with the open approach. Transplantation. 1997;63(2):229–33.
3. Ratner LE, Montgomery RA, Kavoussi LR. Laparoscopic live donor nephrectomy. A review of the first 5 years. Urol Clin N Am. 2001;28(4):709–19.
4. Lee BR, Chow GK, Ratner LE, Kavoussi LR. Laparoscopic live donor nephrectomy: outcomes equivalent to open surgery. J Endourol. 2000;14(10):811–9. discussion 9–20.
5. Rane A, Rao P, Rao P. Single-port-access nephrectomy and other laparoscopic urologic procedures using a novel laparoscopic port (R-port). Urology. 2008;72(2):260–3. discussion 3–4
6. Box G, Averch T, Cadeddu J, Cherullo E, Clayman R, Desai M, et al. Nomenclature of natural orifice translumenal endoscopic surgery (NOTES) and laparoendoscopic single-site surgery (LESS) procedures in urology. J Endourol. 2008;22(11):2575–81.
7. Ganpule AP, Dhawan DR, Kurien A, Sabnis RB, Mishra SK, Muthu V, et al. Laparoendoscopic single-site donor nephrectomy: a single-center experience. Urology. 2009;74(6):1238–40.
8. Richstone L, Rais-Bahrami S, Waingankar N, Hillelsohn JH, Andonian S, Schwartz MJ, et al. Pfannenstiel laparoendoscopic single-site (LESS) vs conventional multiport laparoscopic live donor nephrectomy: a prospective randomized controlled trial. BJU Int. 2013;112(5):616–22.
9. Kurien A, Rajapurkar S, Sinha L, Mishra S, Ganpule A, Muthu V, et al. First prize: standard laparoscopic donor nephrectomy versus laparoendoscopic single-site donor nephrectomy: a randomized comparative study. J Endourol. 2011;25(3):365–70.
10. Autorino R, Brandao LF, Sankari B, Zargar H, Laydner H, Akca O, et al. Laparoendoscopic single-site (LESS) vs laparoscopic living-donor nephrectomy: a systematic review and meta-analysis. BJU Int. 2015;115(2):206–15.
11. Dubey D, Shrinivas RP, Srikanth G. Transumbilical laparoendoscopic single-site donor nephrectomy: without the use of a single port access device. Indian J Urol. 2011;27(2):180–4.
12. Schweitzer EJ, Wilson J, Jacobs S, Machan CH, Philosophe B, Farney A, et al. Increased rates of donation with laparoscopic donor nephrectomy. Ann Surg. 2000;232(3):392–400.

Robotic Donor Nephrectomy

10

Amit S. Bhattu, Arvind P. Ganpule, and Mahesh R. Desai

Abstract

Unlike any other surgery the living donor nephrectomy is a surgery in person who is actually not a patient. Considering the principle of "Primum non nocere" (First do no harm) the responsibility of donor surgeon is highest as it is surgery in person who is not a patient. With this philosophy, the donor surgery evolved from open to laparoscopy and later further modified into robotic assisted laparoscopic living donor nephrectomy (RDN). Robotic platform results in better morbidity profiles for donors than standard laparoscopic approach. It also had advantage in hilar dissection and preservation of longer renal graft artery length in right donor nephrectomy. The graft outcomes of RDN are comparable to LDN. The future development of dedicated robotic single port surgical platforms and instruments as well as multiport approach with transvaginal graft retrieval will be the future direction of development.

Abbreviations

3D	Three dimensional
LDN	Laparoscopic donor nephrectomy
LESS	Laparoendoscopic single-site surgery
HD	High definition
RDN	Robotic-assisted laparoscopic donor nephrectomy
VKD	Living-related voluntary kidney donor

A.S. Bhattu
Jupiter Hospital, Thane, Maharashtra, India

A.P. Ganpule (✉)
Division of Laproscopic and Robotic Surgery, Department of Urology, Muljibhai Patel Urological Hospital, Nadiad, Gujarat, India
e-mail: doctorarvind1@gmail.com

M.R. Desai
Muljbhai Patel Urological Hospital, Dr Virendra Desai Road, Nadiad, Gujarat, India

© Springer Nature Singapore Pte Ltd. 2017
M.R. Desai, A.P. Ganpule (eds.), *Laparoscopic Donor Nephrectomy*,
DOI 10.1007/978-981-10-2849-6_10

113

10.1   Introduction

The optimal and long-term management of end-stage renal disease is renal replacement therapy in the form of renal transplantation. However, the major rate-limiting step in renal transplantation is availability of renal grafts. The deceased donor renal grafts are solution to this in well-developed cadaveric graft retrieval programs. However, the waiting lists in cadaveric graft retrieval programs in developing and developed worlds are significant rate-limiting stage in this aspect. Another alternative in this process is living-related transplantation program with voluntary living-related donors. Moreover, there is some evidence which suggests that the graft outcomes in living-related donor are better than in cadaveric grafts [1, 2].

Unlike any other surgery, the living donor nephrectomy is a surgery in person who is not actually a patient. The donor is a person who has come forward to donate kidney with purely altruistic motive. Considering the principle of "primum non nocere" (first do no harm), the responsibility of donor surgeon is highest as it is surgery in person who is not a patient. Similarly, all attempts should be done to modify the surgery which will minimise the perioperative and postoperative morbidity in donor without compromising on the graft and recipient outcomes. With this philosophy, the donor surgery evolved from open to laparoscopy and later further modified into laparoendoscopic single-site surgery (LESS) and to robotic-assisted laparoscopic living donor nephrectomy (RDN).

In this chapter, we will consider the procedural aspects of the RDN and review the outcomes of this surgery. The preoperative donor workup (medical, ethical and legal) of RDN is same as that of laparoscopic donor nephrectomy.

10.2   Operating Room Setup and Instrumentation

The robotic platform discussed in this chapter is da Vinci Xi or da Vinci Si (Intuitive Surgical®). The da Vinci Si and Xi systems have the following components:

1. *Surgeon console*: Surgeon comfortably sits at console with three-dimensional (3D) high-definition (HD) image within patient's body. Surgeon has master controls below the display, and the hand and fingers are naturally positioned. The movements of the hand, wrist and fingers of surgeon are transmitted in real time to surgical instrument movements within patient body. These instruments are fixed at patient cart.
2. *Patient side cart*: The patient side cart is positioned near patient. It has four arms which pivot around a fixed point. One arm carries the 3D HD camera with corresponding light source, and three arms are for other working instruments. The arms carry out movement as per commands by surgeon at console.
3. *Vision cart*: A HD video of the surgery is available on wide screen to entire operating room and to the bedside surgeon.
4. *Robotic endowrist instruments*: These are the instruments which are attached to the robotic arms and controlled by console surgeon. These instruments have

seven degrees of freedom and precise control from console surgeon. Table 10.1, 10.2 and 10.3. give the details of the instruments required during RDN.

5. *Other robotic instruments* required are as detailed in Table 10.2.
6. *Laparoscopic instrument required*: are detailed in Table 10.3.

10.2.1 Operative Room Setup

The operating room setup is as shown in Fig. 10.1. The robotic surgeons sit on the console. The patient cart is positioned behind the patient. The bedside surgeon and nurse assistant are at patient's side opposite to the patient cart. The nurse assistant

Table 10.1. Robotic endowrist instruments [3]

Instruments	Optional instrument	Use	Preferred arm (the instrument may be shifted from one arm to the other as per requirement)
Monopolar curved scissors	Permanent cautery hook	For bowel reflection and dissection	Right
Maryland bipolar forceps	Fenestrated bipolar forceps or Cardiere forceps	For countertraction during dissection and bowel reflection	Left
ProGrasp forceps	Fenestrated bipolar forceps or Cardiere forceps	For lifting up ureterogonadal packet and/or maintaining inactive countertraction	Fourth arm
Medium-large clip applier (Weck clip)	Laparoscopic Weck clip applier by bedside surgeon	For applying clip to the renal artery or vein or ureter and gonadal vein or any other bleeder	Right
Harmonic ACE curved shears	Laparoscopic harmonic shears by bedside surgeon	For dissection and incising at upper pole of the kidney and other dissection	Right

Table 10.2. Other robotic instruments required in RDN [3]

Instrument	Number
8 mm port cannula	2/3
8 mm port cannula, long	1
8 mm blunt obturator	1
8 mm bladeless obturator	1
8 mm blunt obturator long	1
8 mm bladeless obturator long	1
5–8 mm universal seal to port	3
da Vinci Si (12 mm) or Xi (8 mm) endoscope with camera 30°	1

Table 10.3 Laparoscopic instruments required in RDN

Instruments	Numbers
Veress needle	1
10 mm dilating trocar and ports	3
Suction irrigation system	1
Weck clips medium-large size cartridge	3
Weck clip applier	2
Interlocking clip and applier	1 set with disposable applier
Laparoscopic linear noncutting stapler 45 mm	1
Grasper	1
Maryland forceps	1
Laparoscopic long jaw scissors	1
Laparoscopic Allis forceps	1

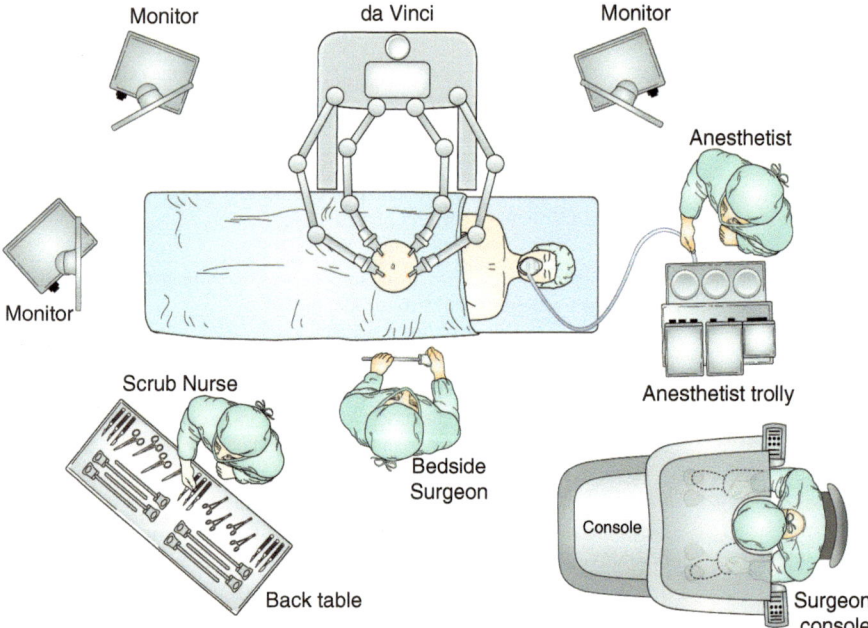

Fig. 10.1 Operative room setup for right RDN

has access to the back trolley of the instruments which are positioned adjacent to him. Anaesthesia team and trolley are at head end of the table. There are multiple HD screens positioned in the operative room which can be seen by bedside surgeons, nurse assistant, anaesthetist and observers. It is important that the screen which bedside surgeon focuses is at his eye level. The robotic arms do not cover any part of this screen even temporarily so that the bedside surgeon has uninterrupted vision of ongoing surgery and is in position to assist efficiently.

10.2.2 Patient Positioning

The surgical table should have good cushioning to ensure that the pressure points are not compressed. Initially living-related voluntary kidney donor (VKD) is positioned in supine position on table. VKD is anaesthetised and intubated with endotracheal tube. VKD is catheterised with Foley catheter 14 Fr under all aseptic precautions, and uro bag is connected to catheter. Uro bag is kept dependent on the bedside surgeon side of the table. The pneumatic compression device is applied to lower limbs of VKD.

Then, the VKD is turned to the lateral decubitus position. The position can be 20 ° less than absolute lateral decubitus position also. For right RDN, the position is left lateral, and for left RDN, it should be right lateral. The abdominal wall of VKD should be at lateral edge of the table. After turning the patient, it is ensured by anaesthetist that the endotracheal tube is properly positioned and monitor probes are properly connected. Surgical team ensures that the Foley catheter and tubing are not compressed and draining urine freely.

The back of the VKD is supported with cushioned packs. The position of inferior lower limb of patient is important. The contralateral limb (left lower limb in case of right RDN and right lower limb in case of left LDN) should be flexed at the knee and positioned in such a way that the knee should not project beyond the edge of the table as this may restrict the movement of instrument and bedside surgeon working space. The ipsilateral lower limb (left in case of left LDN and right in case of right LDN) should be in complete extension position. A cushion is placed between the lower limbs.

Few centres recommend extension of kidney bridge for increasing the distance between the ipsilateral iliac crest and subcostal margin. Theoretically, this may assist the dissection, but at our centre, we did not find this manoeuvre necessary as the pneumoperitoneum itself creates enough space for dissection. However, as discussed later in the procedure part, if the movement of fourth arm is getting restricted, then the table may be extended to raise the kidney bridge. Once positioning of patient is acceptable, then the straps are put at nipple level and at buttock level of the patient with sufficient padding to prevent pressure injury. The straps at nipple level should be loose enough to allow the respiratory excursion. This can be achieved by placing surgeon's hand on lateral aspect of chest over which the straps are tightened.

10.3   Right RDN

It is advisable to do surface marking prior to the port placement at least in early learning curve. The midline of abdominal wall should be marked. The lateral wall of the rectus should be marked. Anterior superior iliac spine, iliac crest, subcostal margin and 11th rib tip should be marked. These surface markings allow the orientation to be maintained during the port placement.

A small 2 mm stab is done on ipsilateral midpoint of spinoumbilical line, and pneumoperitoneum is induced with Veress needle (Fig. 10.2). The approximate relation of renal hilum in reference to 11th rib is noted with help of renal CT angiography which is done as preoperative workup. The fist port is camera port. It is 12 mm dilating port placed at lateral border of rectus at level of renal hilum (Fig. 10.3). Laparoscopy is done and the abdominal cavity is reviewed for adhesions at the abdominal wall, bleeding if any into peritoneal cavity during port placement or at time of Veress needle insertion. It is reinsured that there are no adhesions at Pfannenstiel incision site which is proposed site of retrieval incision. This is particularly important post-Caesarian sections and gynaecological surgeries.

Pfannenstiel incision is marked and incision is deepened through the skin and subcutaneous tissue (Fig. 10.4). The anterior rectus sheath is incised transversely and both recti are seen. Pneumoperitoneum is deflated and plane is created between anterior rectus sheath and recti cranially as well as caudally sufficient enough to allow the

Fig. 10.2 Induction of pneumoperitoneum

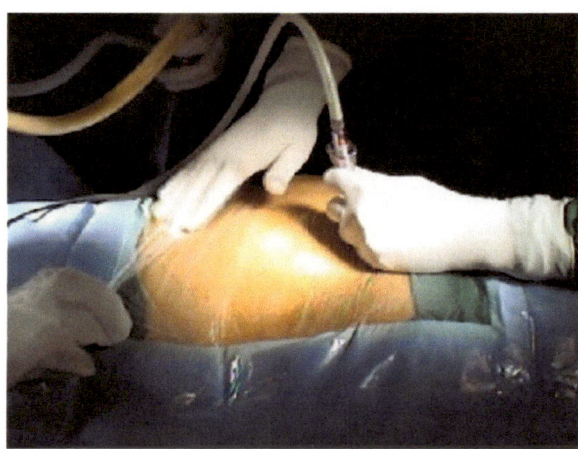

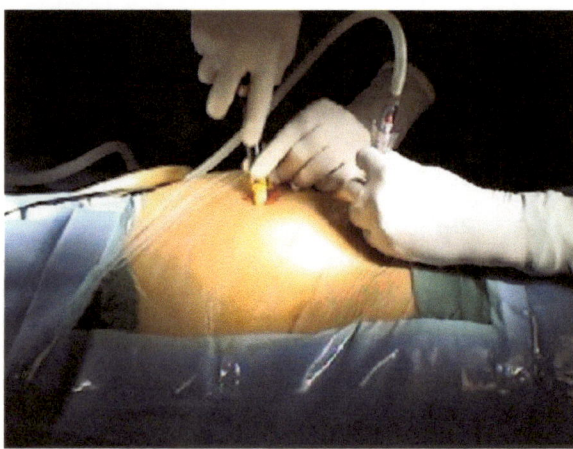

Fig. 10.3 Placement of first port

Fig. 10.4 Pfannenstiel
incision placement

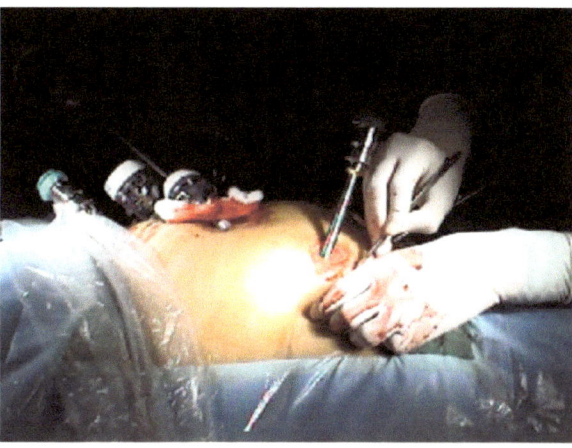

lateral retraction of recti. Both recti are retracted away from each other laterally, and properitoneal pad of fat is noted. The pneumoperitoneum is reinduced; it helps in proper dissection of properitoneal pad of fat and visualisation of parietal peritoneum. After careful dissection, transparent parietal peritoneum is noted which is preserved for incision at the time of final graft retrieval. These steps are necessary to ensure that the retrieval is fast and warm ischaemia time is minimum, and it is to be insisted that care has to be taken not to damage the parietal peritoneum at this time because it may lead to the leaking of pneumoperitoneum throughout the procedure.

Just like in laparoscopic surgery, the appropriate port placement is important in robotic surgery as well, but it is not as critical in robotic surgery. However, the care has to be taken in robotic surgery to ensure that the ports are at least four finger-breadths away from each other in inflated abdominal wall. This is necessary for ensuring the proper functioning of robotic arms. If the ports are very closely placed, the clashing of robotic arms compromises its manoeuvrability.

One 8 mm robotic port is placed just below the subcostal border at the level of or little lateral to the mid-clavicular line. This is port for right robotic arm. Another 8 mm robotic port is placed few centimetres lateral to the midpoint of the spinoumbilical line. This is port for left robotic arm. The port used for fourth arm should be 8 mm long metal port; it is placed cranial and lateral to ipsilateral end of Pfannenstiel incision, and it should be caudal and medial to the midpoint of the spinoumbilical line. This port should be long port so that the fourth arm can be manoeuvred easily. If there is difficulty in manoeuvrability of fourth arm after docking, then as discussed earlier, the table may be broken to raise the kidney bridge or to lower the lower limbs of patient. It is necessary to ensure that the robotic fourth arm does not directly put pressure over patient's lower limb.

Additional bedside surgeon working port is placed medial and cranial to the camera port. It should be 12 mm dilating port (Fig. 10.5).

Five millimetre port is placed in the midline or on the left side of midline below the xiphisternum for inserting the Allis forceps for liver retraction. Allis forceps is passed through this port fixed to lateral aspect of the diaphragmatic muscles to

Fig. 10.5 Final port
placement

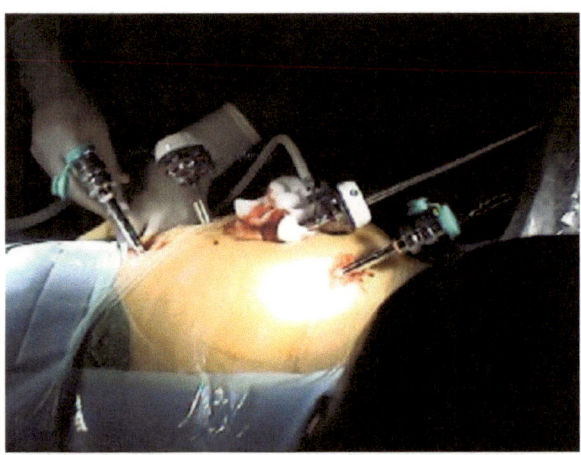

Fig. 10.6 Liver retraction
port

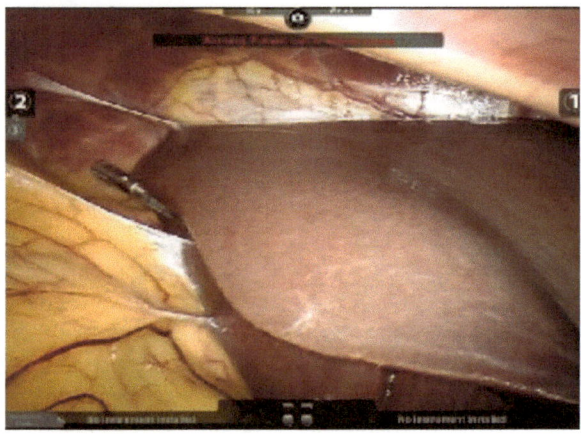

ensure good liver retraction. This is done after releasing adhesion of inferior border
of liver surface if there are any (Fig. 10.6).

Another 12 mm dilating port is placed from Pfannenstiel incision through the
ipsilateral rectus sheath and muscle. This port is for insertion of vascular stapler for
clamping the graft renal vein.

Then the motorised patient cart is moved towards the patient, and the robotic
arms are connected to corresponding robotic ports and camera port (Fig. 10.7), taking care of fourth arm as described above. After connecting the robotic camera in
camera port, all the robotic instruments are inserted and docked under vision to
ensure that the instrument is inserted in correct path without damaging any intervening structure.

Right robotic instrument monopolar curved scissors are inserted and connected
to the monopolar cautery. Left robotic arm instrument is Maryland forceps, and it is
connected to bipolar cautery (Fig. 10.8). Fourth arm instrument is ProGrasp forceps. Robot is docked, and now the console surgeon starts operating from console.

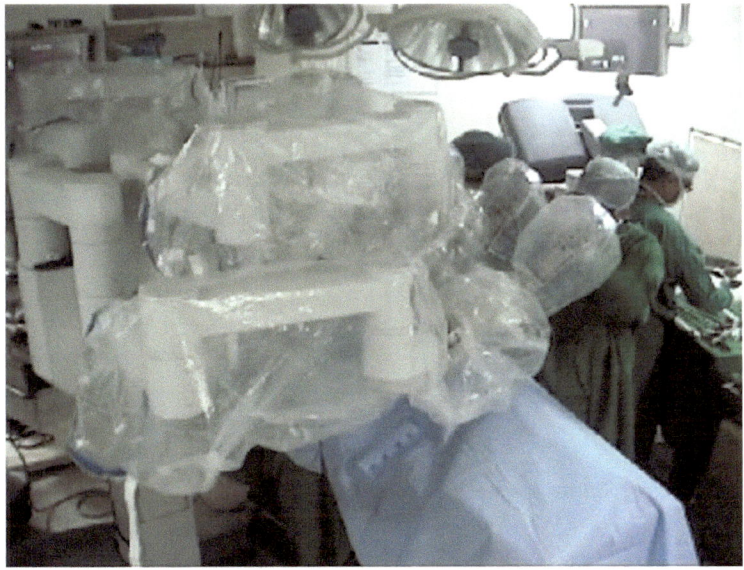

Fig. 10.7 Robotic docking

Fig. 10.8 Insertion of robotic instruments

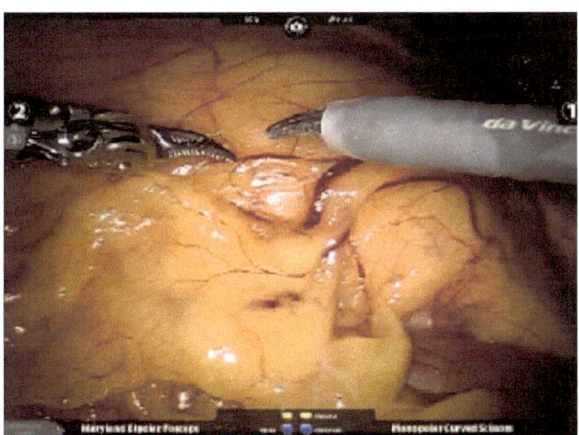

The reflection of ascending colon: A plane is developed between the peritoneal fat and surface of Gerota's fascia by holding the parietal peritoneum lateral to the ascending colon with maryland forceps and gently giving traction over it. The fibro-fatty tissue in this plane is incised with monopolar curved scissor, and the ascending colon is reflected. The same plane is followed up to the pelvic brim, and the whole anterior Gerota's fascia surface is exposed.

Now the inferior vena cava (IVC) can be seen in inferior aspect of the field; however, the renal hilum is still covered with the duodenum. The duodenum is Kocherised by incising the parietal peritoneal layer lateral to the duodenum with sharp cold cut with monopolar curved scissor (Fig. 10.9).

Fig. 10.9 Kocherisation of duodenum

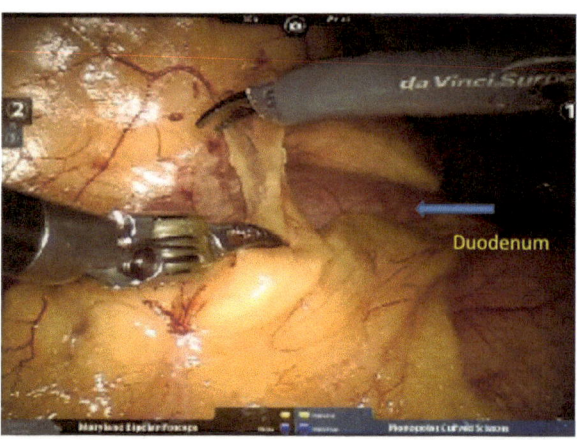

Fig. 10.10 Right gonadal vein draining into inferior vena cava

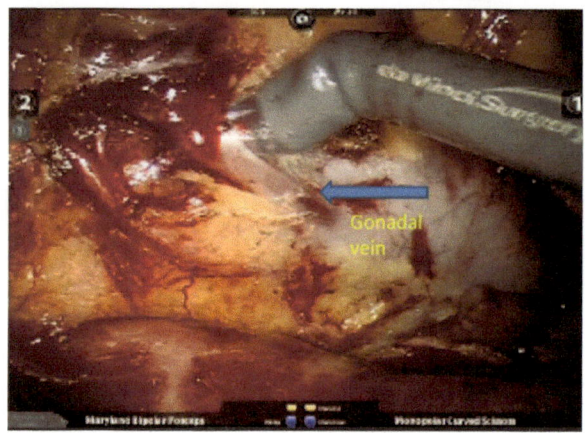

Now IVC forms the horizon. With blunt and sharp dissection, the anterior Gerota's fascia is incised just lateral to IVC, and ureterogonadal packet is lifted up over the psoas sheath. At this stage, care should be taken not to enter the psoas sheath. Plane should be developed over the psoas sheath, and the gonadal vein as well as ureter is lifted up in one packet without dissecting around the ureter to preserve the ureteric vascularity.

After lifting up, the ureter is kept lifted up to with ProGrasp forceps in fourth arm. If console surgeon feels necessary, the instruments in fourth arm and left arm are switched and ProGrasp is used to keep the ureter lifted up.

Now with ureterogonadal packet lifted up, the blunt and sharp dissection is continued cranially. The gonadal vein draining into the IVC is noted at this stage (Fig. 10.10). The gonadal vein is doubly clipped with Weck clips with two clips towards IVC and one clip towards the gonadal vein; the gonadal vein is transected (Fig. 10.11). The Weck clips are either applied by console surgeon with robotic

Fig. 10.11 Clipping of right gonadal vein

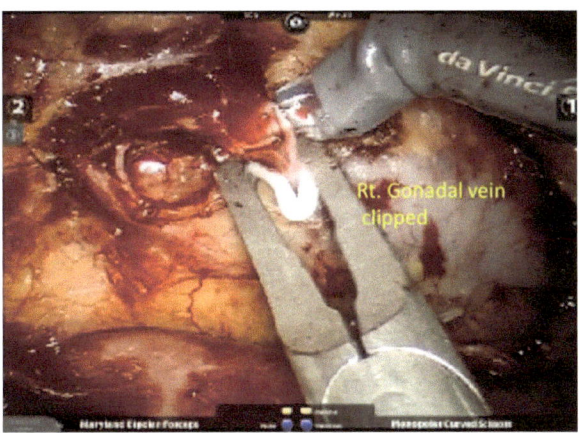

week clip applier or it can also be applied by bedside surgeon. At our centre, the Weck clips are applied by bedside surgeon as it saves time which is spent in robotic instrument change, and multiple laparoscopic clip applier can be kept ready for quickly applying multiple clips. This particularly becomes relevant in hilar vessel clipping as that time accounts for warm ischaemia time.

After the gonadal vein is clipped, further cranial dissection reaches the hilar level. With prior study of renal CT angiography, the number of arteries and veins and their relative positions and level of branching are known before the surgery. By lifting the ureterogonadal packet, the branching points of the artery are more lateral than as seen in the CT; this adds favourably to surgeon comfort and getting better artery length.

The challenges in right renal hilar dissections are short right renal vein and right lumbar vein directly draining into IVC behind the renal vein which may be the source of bleeding and right renal artery dissection which may need retrocaval dissection [4]. The robotic platform with its 3D HD vision, seven degrees of freedom and tremor filter facilitates these steps [5]. During hilar dissection, the fibrofatty tissues between the artery and vein including the lymphatics should be cleared. The artery and vein should be skeletonising (Fig. 10.12). Longer artery length can be achieved with retrocaval dissection. Robotic camera can also allow good view of retrocaval area and the posterior aspect of right renal vein. The right lumbar vein may be entering the IVC near this area. To achieve longer artery length, the retrocaval dissection may also be facilitated by complete flipping of the kidney after releasing the upper pole and lateral attachment of the graft.

Once the hilar dissection is done, upper pole dissection is initiated. With the help of monopolar curved scissor or with harmonic shear, the dissection is continued intragerotaly at the upper pole. Adrenal gland is carefully preserved in donor, and upper pole is freed completely.

Now intravascular mannitol is given by anaesthetist with good hydration maintained all throughout the procedure. The papaverine in 1:10 normal saline dilution is injected over the surface of hilar vessels.

Fig. 10.12 Appearance
after skeletonising graft
artery and vein

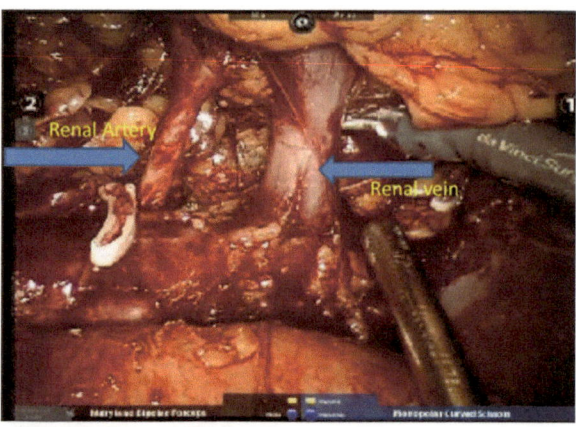

Fig. 10.13 Gonadal vein
clipping

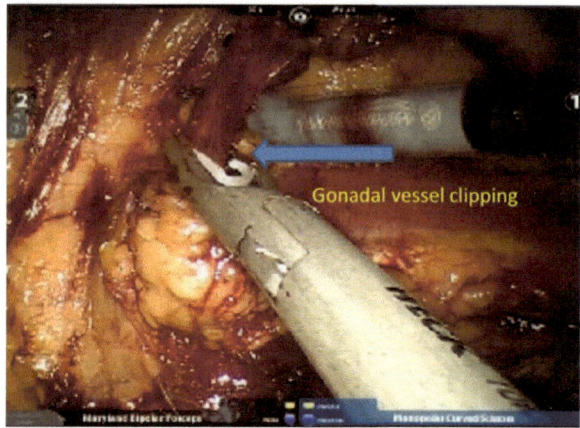

Gonadal vein is now dissected in ureterogonadal packet; it is doubly clipped with Weck clip and transected (Fig. 10.13). Ureter is identified again, but it is not skeletonised to preserve its vascularity. Ureter is clipped distally at the pelvic brim with Weck clip and cut proximal to clip (Fig. 10.14). Good efflux of urine from the cut end of ureter is confirmed. Now the lateral attachments of the Gerota's fascia are incised to preserve only minimal attachment just lateral to the kidney to keep the kidney hanging from the lateral side for facilitating the hilar clamping and transection of the hilar vessels.

Now the renal artery is clipped with two Weck clips and transected keeping minimum 1 mm renal artery cuff distal to distal clip over the donor side, preserving maximum possible length of graft artery. This can be done either by robotic clip applier or laparoscopic week clip applier by bedside surgeon. As discussed earlier in this text, Weck clips are applied by bedside surgeon at our centre, and graft artery is transected by robotic console surgeon with robotic curved scissors. Similarly, the

Fig. 10.14 Ureteric clipping

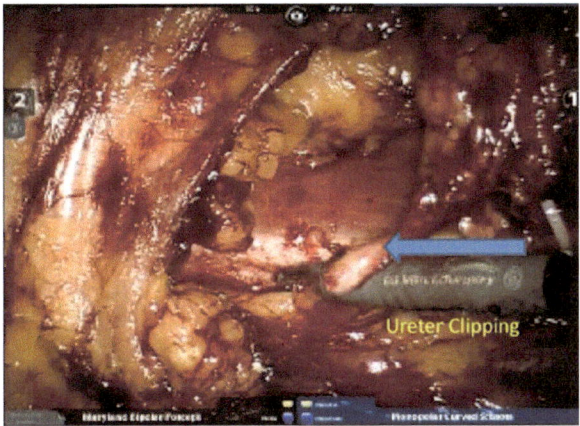

Fig. 10.15 Securing the graft vein with vascular stapler

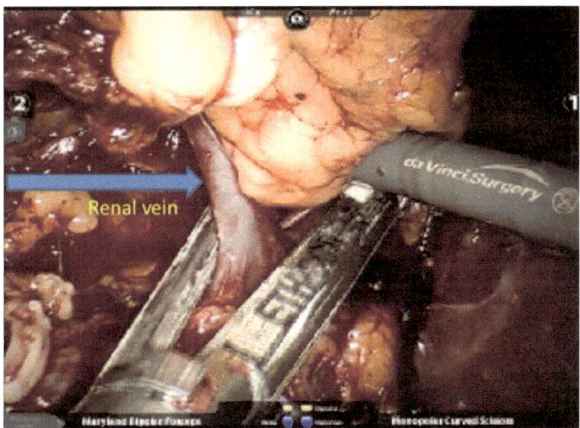

renal vein can be clipped with two Weck clips towards the donor side, and the vein is cut 1 mm distal to distal clip preserving maximum possible length of graft vein. However, at our centre, considering the short and broad nature of right renal vein, the right renal vein is secured with laparoscopic linear noncutting stapler 45 mm which is passed through the 12 mm dilating port placed through the Pfannenstiel incision (Fig. 10.15). The console surgeon cuts the vein distal to the staple line with robotic scissor (Fig. 10.16).

Now the console surgeon incises all the lateral attachments of the graft, and graft is placed free in the renal fossa (Fig. 10.17). All the robotic instruments grips are released so that instruments are not holding any donor tissues. Bedside surgeon now removes the instruments in third (left) and fourth arm and undocks the third (left) and fourth robotic arms. The parietal peritoneum in the Pfannenstiel incision is sharply incised. The port in Pfannenstiel incision is removed. Bedside surgeon now puts his hand in the peritoneal cavity through the incision and removes the third and

Fig. 10.16 Transection of graft renal vein proximal to stapler line

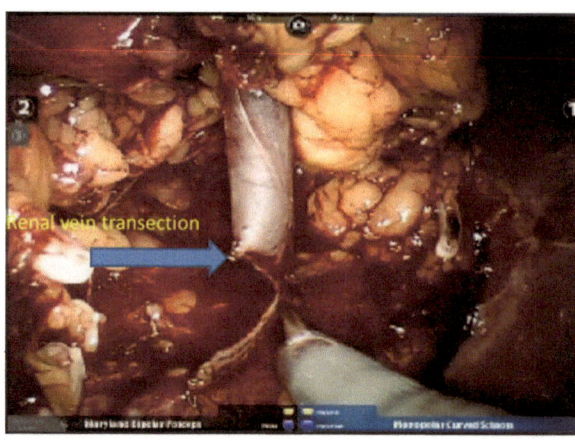

Fig. 10.17 Release of lateral attachment of graft

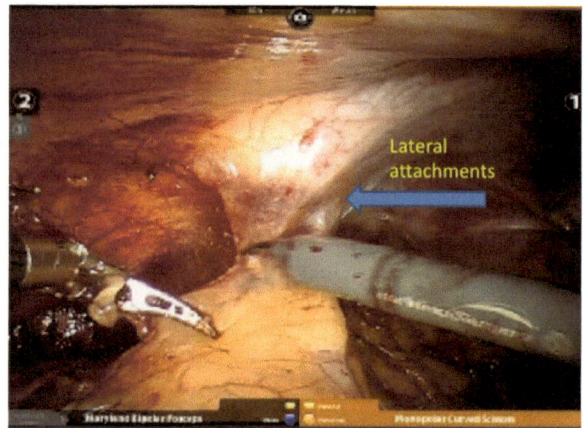

fourth arm ports temporarily if necessary. The renal graft which is placed free in the right renal fossa is retrieved through the wound in longitudinal axis and delivered to the bench surgeon who immediately perfuses the graft. Now the rest of the robotic arms are undocked.

Check laparoscopy is done with donor surgeon's hand sealing the Pfannenstiel wound to check for any active bleeding. Then the Pfannenstiel wound is closed in layers. Formal check laparoscopy is done now to check for active oozing or chylous leaking. Haemostasis is achieved with cautery or with Weck clips or interlocking clips. Suspected lymphatics are clipped with Weck clips. Liberal warm saline peritoneal wash is given with suction irrigation cannula to wash away the blood and urine which has drained into the peritoneal cavity after ureteric transection. Liver-retracting Allis forceps is released. Twelve millimetre ports are closed with Carter-Thomason II Port Closure System. Drain placement is never required.

10.4   Left RDN

The surface marking, induction of pneumoperitoneum and port placement and Pfannenstiel incision placement and robotic docking are similar in left LDN as in right LDN (Figs. 10.18, 10.19, 10.20 and 10.21) other than the following differences:

- The 12 mm dilating port in Pfannenstiel incision which is placed in right RDN is not required in left RDN.
- Liver retraction port is not required on the left side.
- The left subcostal port is for left arm instruments.
- The monopolar curved scissor is put from right arm port, and it comes from the cranial and lateral to the midpoint of spinoumbilical line.
- The fourth arm which comes craniolateral to the left edge of Pfannenstiel incision is for ProGrasp as on the right side.

Fig. 10.18 Induction of pneumoperitoneum

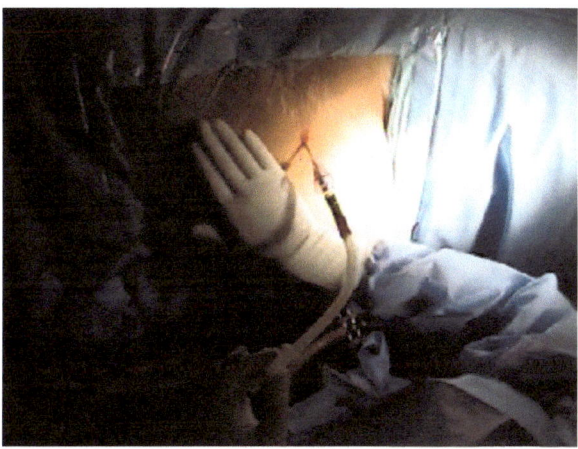

Fig. 10.19 Placement of first port

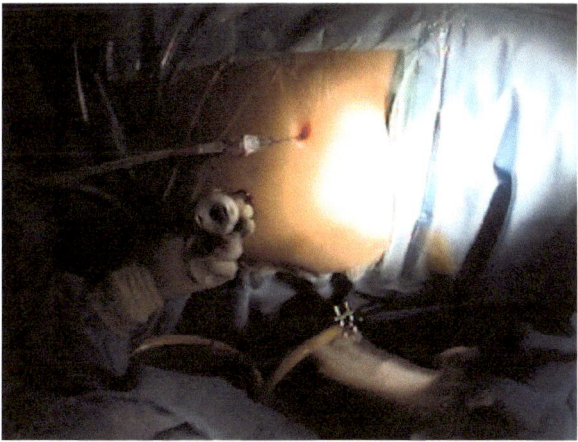

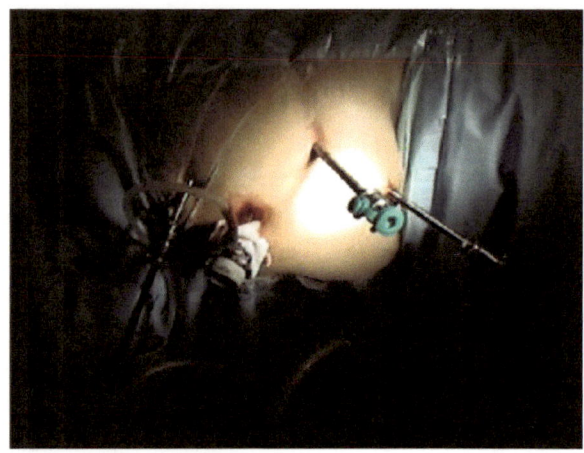

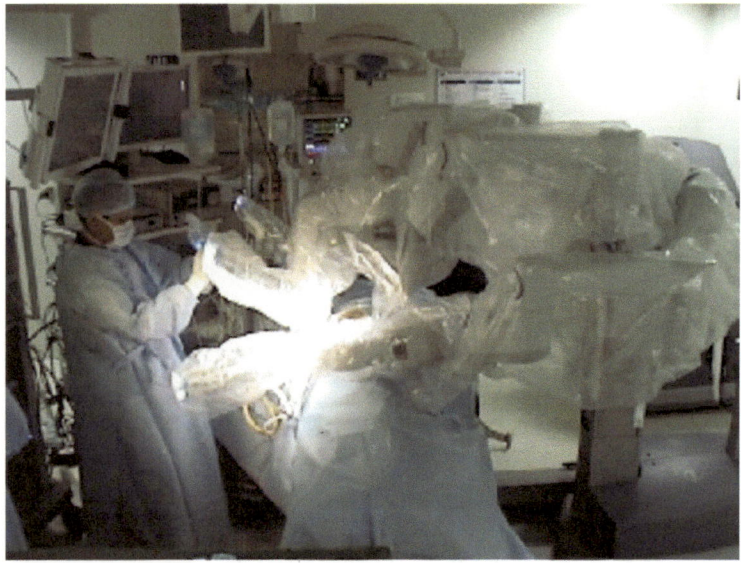

Fig. 10.21 Robotic docking

The reflection of the bowel is started from white line of Toldt (Fig. 10.22). The descending colon is reflected, and plane is achieved at anterior Gerota's fascia level (Fig. 10.23). Then the ureterogonadal packet is lifted up over the psoas sheath and kept lifted up with ProGrasp forceps (Figs. 10.24 and 10.25). The dissection is continued cranially, and the descending colon is completely reflected to identify the anterior surface of the left renal vein. Now the lateral border of the aorta should be seen as horizon craniocaudally, and seeing the abdominal aorta craniocaudally also confirms the adequate reflection of descending colon.

Fig. 10.22 Incision on white line of Toldt

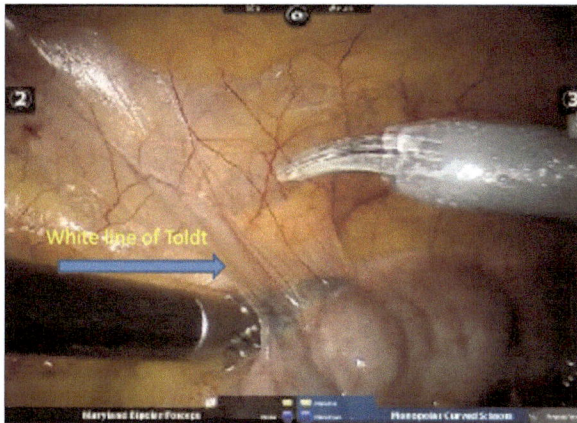

Fig. 10.23 Dissection at anterior Gerota's fascia level after reflection of descending colon

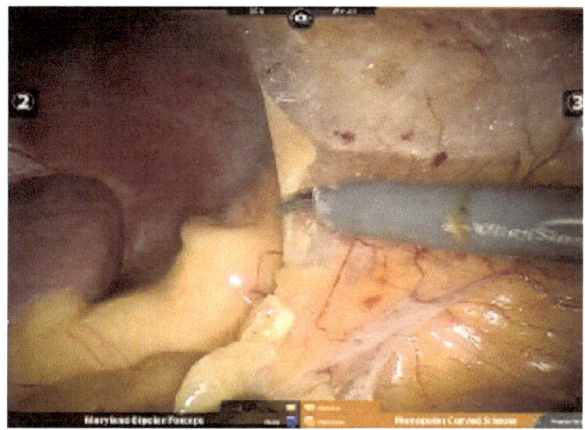

Now the dissection is continued at the cranial boarder of the left renal vein to identify the insertion of the left adrenal vein into the left renal vein. Once the left adrenal vein is identified, it is dissected cranially till sufficient length of adrenal vein is exposed (Fig. 10.26). The adrenal vein is doubly clipped with and cut between the clips (Figs. 10.27 and 10.28). The dissection now is proceeded towards the upper pole and with harmonic shear or with monopolar curved scissors. The adrenal gland is separated from the upper pole of the kidney, and then the dissection is continued till complete release and cutting of lienorenal ligament (Fig. 10.29). This completes the upper polar dissection.

Now focus is moved to renal hilum. With permanent cautery hook or with monopolar curved scissors, the perihilar fat is dissected with 30° camera positioned to see craniolaterally and posterior to the renal vein from lower border of the renal vein. The left lumbar vein will be encountered first at this stage which is skeletonised and clipped and cut between the clips (Figs. 10.30 and 10.31). After

Fig. 10.24 Lifting up of ureterogonadal packet

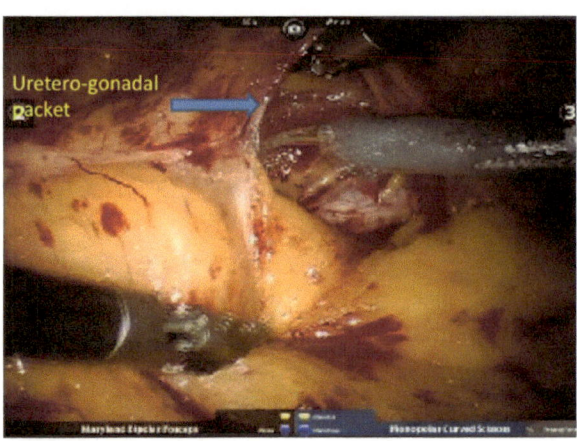

Fig. 10.25 Lifting up of ureterogonadal packet

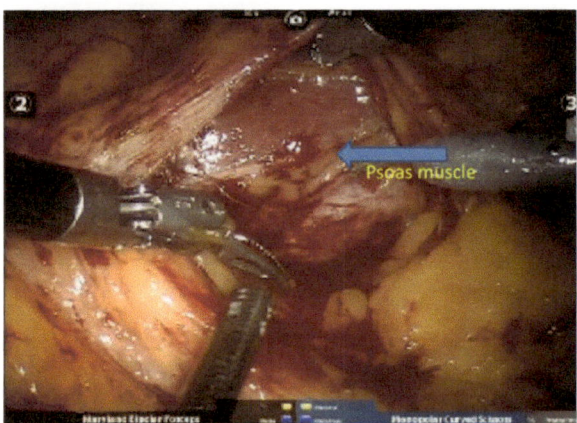

Fig. 10.26 Dissection of left adrenal vein

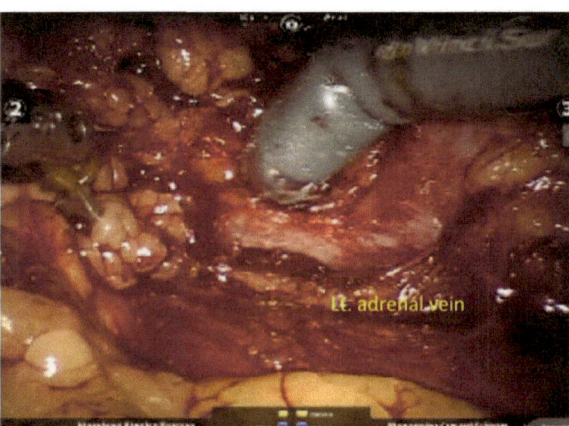

Fig. 10.27 Clipping and transection of left adrenal vein

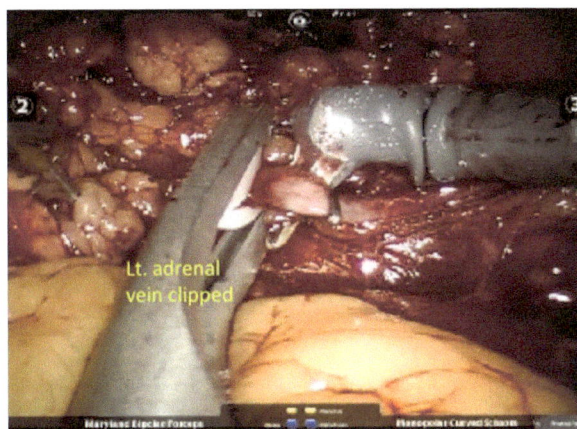

Fig. 10.28 Clipping and transection of left adrenal vein

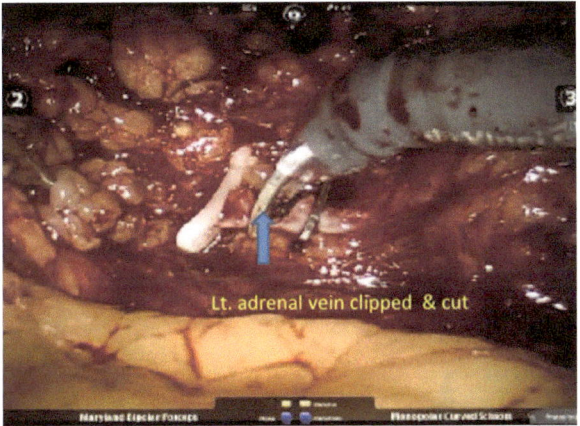

Fig. 10.29 Left upper pole dissection

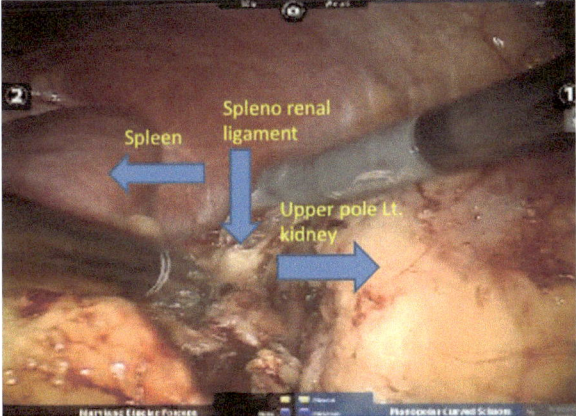

Fig. 10.30 Clipping of
left lumbar vein

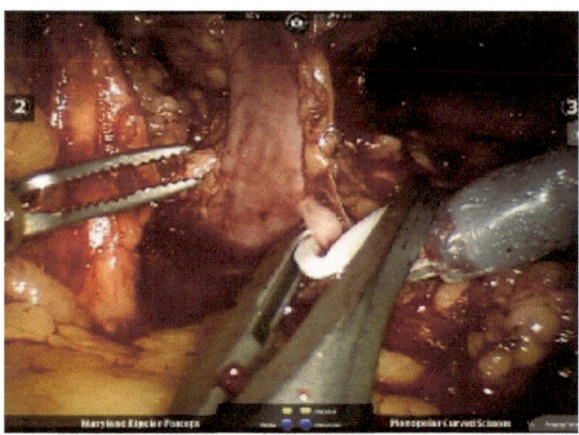

Fig. 10.31 Transection
left lumbar vein

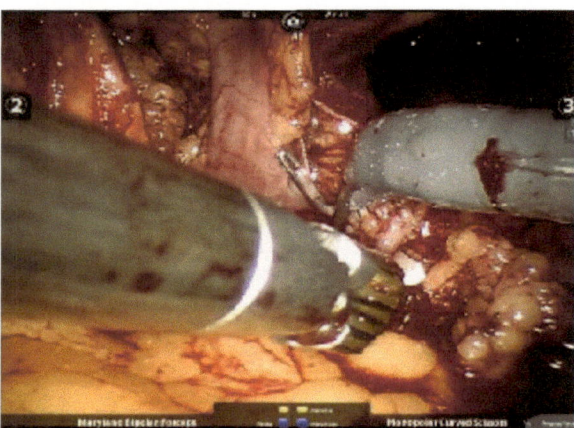

transection of the lumbar vein, the renal vein further straightens up, and further dissection posterior to the renal vein will show the left renal artery. The relative positions of the left renal vein and artery are already known by preoperative review of the renal CT angiography. The renal artery and vein are skeletonised at this stage (Fig. 10.32). If felt necessary, a sling is passed around the graft artery, and with gentle traction over the sling, the dissection is facilitated (Fig. 10.33). The renal artery origin from the aorta is noted, and this is the site where the Weck clip will be applied later to preserve the maximal left renal artery length. The papaverine injection in 1:10 dilution is normal saline which is injected over the surface of hilar vessels.

The ureterogonadal dissection and transection of the ureter and gonadal vein is similar to right side (Figs. 10.34, 10.35, 10.36 and 10.37). Now as on right side, the lateral attachments of the left kidney are reduced and kept just enough to keep the left kidney hanging from the lateral side.

Fig. 10.32 Hilar vessel
dissection

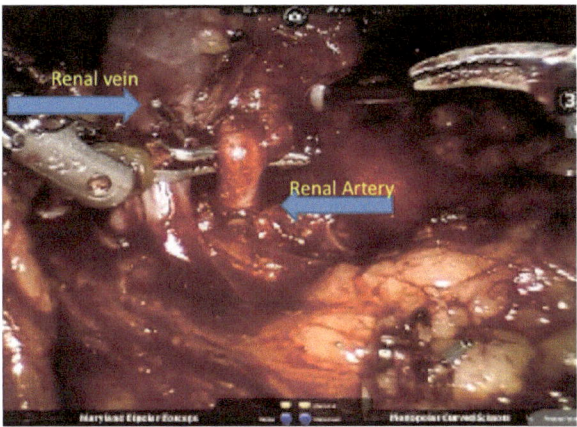

Fig. 10.33 Slinging the
graft artery for facilitating
hilar dissection

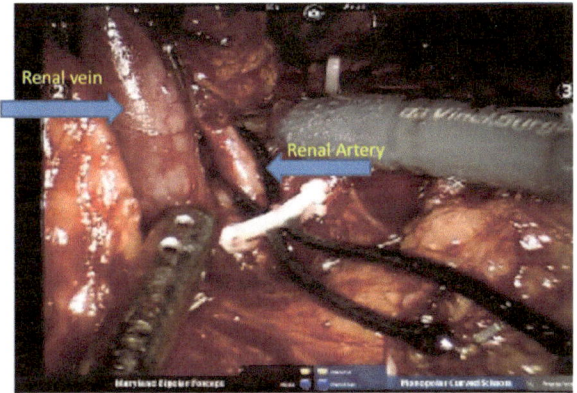

Fig. 10.34 Clipping of
left gonadal vein

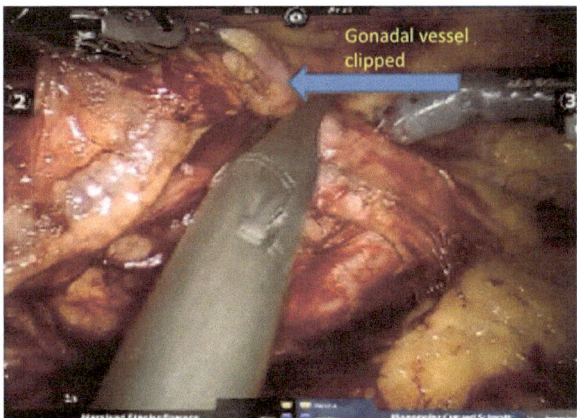

Fig. 10.35 Transection of left gonadal vein

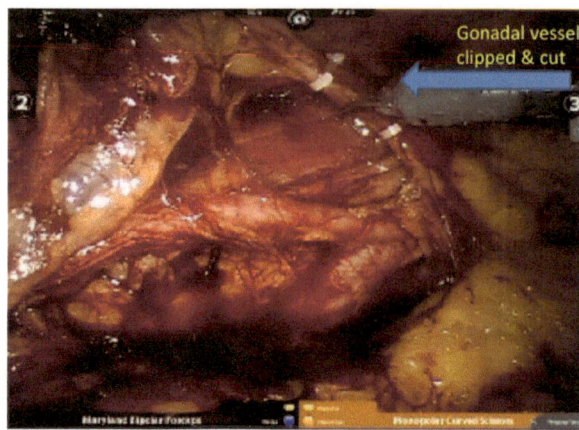

Fig. 10.36 Clipping of left ureter

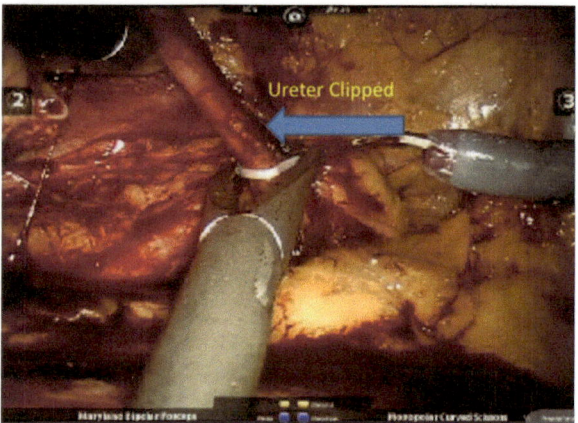

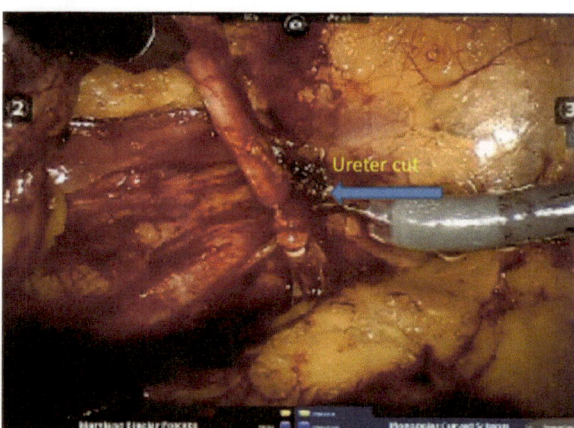

Fig. 10.37 Transection of left ureter

Now again focus is moved to renal hilum. The left renal artery is doubly clipped with Weck clips just distal to its origin (Fig. 10.38). The renal artery is transected keeping 1 mm cuff distal to distal Weck clip (Fig. 10.39). Then, the renal vein is doubly clipped with Weck clip and transected proximal (graft side of the week clip keeping 1 mm cuff) keeping maximum left renal vein length possible (Figs. 10.40 and 10.41).

The lateral attachments of the left kidney are released, and graft is placed free in the left renal fossa. All the robotic instruments grips are released so that instruments are not holding any donor tissues. Bedside surgeon now removes the instruments in first (right) and fourth arm and undocks the first (right) and fourth robotic arms. The parietal peritoneum in the Pfannenstiel incision is sharply incised. Bedside surgeon now puts his hand in the peritoneal cavity through the incision and removes the first and fourth arm ports temporarily if necessary. The renal graft which is placed free in the left renal fossa is retrieved through the wound in longitudinal axis and delivered to the bench surgeon who immediately perfuses the graft. Now the rest of the robotic arms are undocked.

Fig. 10.38 Clipping of left renal graft artery

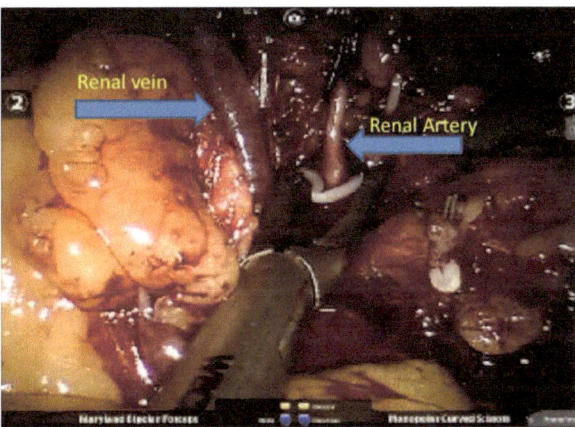

Fig. 10.39 Transection of left renal graft artery

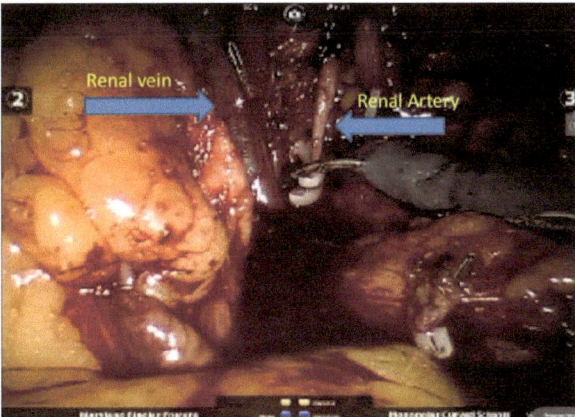

Check laparoscopy and port closure are done as mentioned in right RDN after closure of Pfannenstiel incision (Fig. 10.42).

10.5   Review of Literature

Horgan and team reported first series of ten cases of RDN in 2002 [6]. They reported better precision, better hand-eye coordination, more comfort and equally good early outcomes in RDN compared to laparoscopic donor nephrectomy (LDN).

Literature suggests that robotic approach is associated with lesser pain compared to laparoscopic approach [7]. In robotic surgery, the robotic arms which are pivoted around port site are moved around fixed remote centre. This leads to lesser leverage and pressure at port site and less stretching at port site which leads to lesser pain compared to laparoscopic surgery.

Randomised controlled trial comparing RDN and LDN [5] suggested that RDN is associated with less postoperative pain, analgesic requirements and hospital stay

Fig. 10.40 Clipping of left renal graft vein

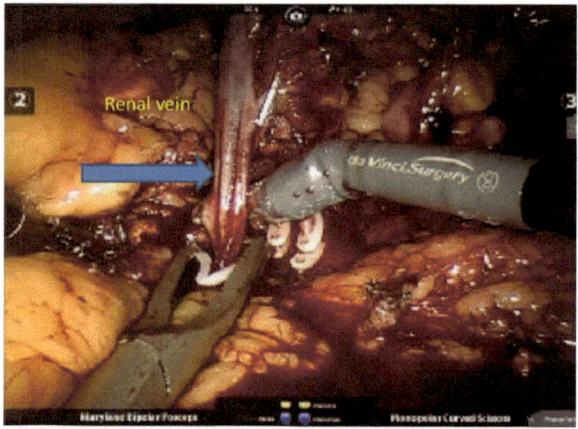

Fig. 10.41 Transection of left renal graft vein

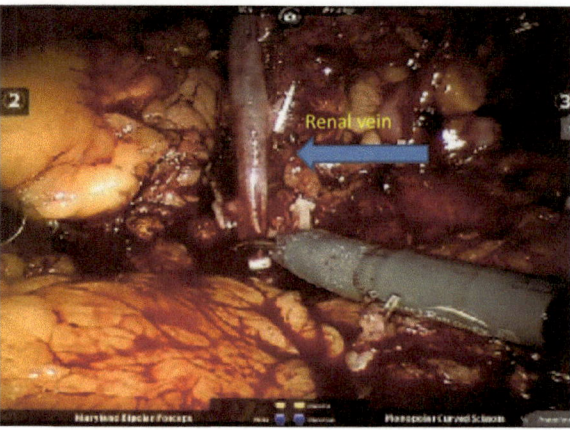

Fig. 10.42 Check laparoscopy

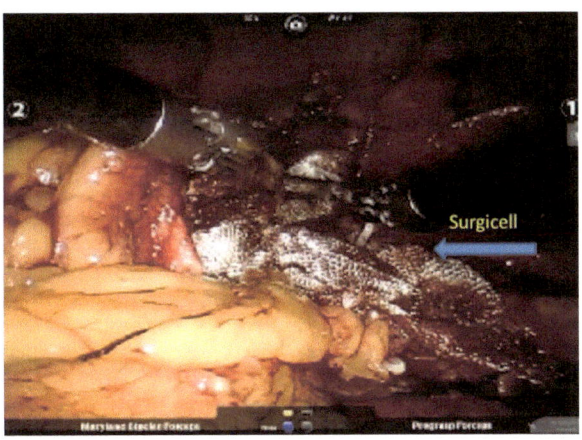

in RDN group. The RDN is as safe as LDN, and there were no donor complications in the study in any group. There was no conversion from RDN to LDN or to open donor nephrectomy in any patient. The graft outcome in RDN and LDN groups was comparable up to 9-month follow-up. There was no difference in donor's total operative time, haemoglobin drop or serum creatinine at 1 month in both the groups. More number of ports were required in RDN than LDN. Graft retrieval time was longer in RDN than LDN. The left RDN had higher warm ischaemia time than left LDN; however, there was no significant difference in warm ischaemia time between right RDN and LDN. Longer graft artery length can be preserved in right RDN by achieving better retrocaval right renal artery dissection than right LDN; however, there was no significant difference in preserved artery length between left RDN and LDN. There was no significant difference in preserved vein length between RDN and LDN on either side. In RDN, two surgeons were required (one on patient side and another on console), whereas in LDN single laparoscopic surgeon is required. In right RDN, the reported difficulty score (VAS) of console surgeon was less than right LDN surgeon at all stages except at stage of upper pole dissection which had similar VAS scores. The VAS score of console surgeon in left RDN was less than VAS score of left LDN surgeon only in step of renal artery and vein transection; for all other steps of surgery, it was similar. The VAS score of bedside surgeon was more for retrieval of graft in RDN than LDN on either side. This was related to undocking of robotic arms required at the stage of retrieval. This is also the reason for more retrieval time in RDN compared to LDN.

Literature suggests that the use of robotic approach increases the cost of treatment for donor surgery [8]. However, it is also suggested that robotic approach decreases hospital stay and hence will eventually lead to decreased cost of treatment [4, 9].

LESS is technically demanding approach, and hence its application in donor nephrectomy is challenging. A case report describing robotic LESS donor nephrectomy reports of improving the ease associated with LESS donor nephrectomy and proposes that this approach through single small incision may provide better cosmesis, lesser pain, early recovery and possibly better acceptance of donor nephrectomy [10].

Case reports also describe combining the RDN with transvaginal extraction of graft. These reports claim faster recovery due to absence of retrieval incision on abdominal wall and better cosmesis [11].

To summarise, robotic platform resulted in better morbidity profiles for donors than standard laparoscopic approach in present studies. It also had advantage in hilar dissection and preservation of longer renal graft artery length in right donor nephrectomy. The graft outcomes of RDN are comparable to LDN. The future development of dedicated robotic single-port surgical platforms and instruments as well as multi-port approach with transvaginal graft retrieval will be the future direction of development.

References

1. Schulam PG et al. Laparoscopic live donor nephrectomy: the initial 3 cases. J Urol. 1996;155:1857–9.
2. Cecka JM. The UNOS Scientific renal transplant registry–2000. Clin Transpl. 2000:1–8.
3. da Vinci Xi instrument and accessory catalogue: May 2015.
4. Ahlawat RK. Commentary on Transperitoneal laparoscopic left versus right live donor nephrectomy: Comparison of outcomes. Indian J Urol. 2014;30:261–2.
5. Bhattu AS, Ganpule A, Sabnis RB, Murali V, Mishra S, Desai M. Robot-assisted laparoscopic donor nephrectomy vs standard laparoscopic donor nephrectomy: a prospective randomized comparative study. J Endourol. 2015;29(12):1334–40.
6. Horgan S, Vanuno D, Sileri P, Cicalese L, Benedetti E. Robotic-assisted laparoscopic donor nephrectomy for kidney transplantation. Transplantation. 2002;73:1474–9.
7. Chiu LH, Chen CH, Tu PC, Chang CW, Yen YK, Liu WM. Comparison of robotic surgery and laparoscopy to perform total hysterectomy with pelvic adhesions or large uterus. J Minimal Access Surg. 2015;11:87–93.
8. Monn MF, Gramm AR, Bahler CD, Yang DY, Sundaram CP. Economic and utilization analysis of robot-assisted versus laparoscopic live donor nephrectomy. J Endourol. 2014;28:780–3.
9. Cohen AJ, Williams DS, Bohorquez H, et al. Robotic-assisted laparoscopic donor nephrectomy: decreasing length of stay. Ochsner J. 2015;15:19–24.
10. Galvani CA, Garza U, Leeds M, et al. Single-incision robotic-assisted living donor nephrectomy: case report and description of surgical technique. Transpl Int. 2012;25(8):e89–92.
11. Pietrabissa A, Abelli M, Spinillo A, et al. Robotic-assisted laparoscopic donor nephrectomy with transvaginal extraction of the kidney. Am J Transplant. 2010;10(12):2708–11.

T.A. Kishore

Abstract

Laparoscopy has become the standard method for donor kidney extraction, since 1995 [1]. Graft extraction is one of the most critical steps in living donor nephrectomy. Extraction incision plays an important role in patient outcome. It has an impact on post-operative pain, wound complications and cosmesis. Moreover the process of extraction is a time-sensitive technique and can have a impact on ultimate graft function. Unlike other ablative laparoscopic procedures, it is imperative that the kidney has to be extracted without any damage to the graft. The extent and location of the incision can concede the inherent advantage laparoscopic procedures possess over the open technique. Over the years, surgeons have resorted to various techniques of extraction to reduce the morbidity and improve the safety profile.

11.1 Introduction

Laparoscopy has become the standard method for donor kidney extraction, since 1995 [1]. Graft extraction is one of the most critical steps in living donor nephrectomy. Extraction incision plays an important role in patient outcome. It has an impact on post-operative pain, wound complications and cosmesis. Moreover the process of extraction is a time-sensitive technique and can impact on ultimate graft function. Unlike other ablative laparoscopic procedures, it is imperative that the kidney has to be extracted without any damage to the graft. The extent and location

T.A. Kishore
Aster Medcity,
Kuttisahib Road, Near Kothad Bridge South Chittoor P. O, Cheranelloor, Kochi 682027,
Kerala, India
e-mail: kishoreta@yahoo.com

© Springer Nature Singapore Pte Ltd. 2017
M.R. Desai, A.P. Ganpule (eds.), *Laparoscopic Donor Nephrectomy*,
DOI 10.1007/978-981-10-2849-6_11

of the incision can concede the inherent advantage laparoscopic procedures possess over the open technique. Over the years, surgeons have resorted to various techniques of extraction to reduce the morbidity and improve the safety profile. Hand-assisted and pure laparoscopic methods were the popular methods in the last decade, and recently, few authors have also reported single-port techniques [2–6].

Various techniques of graft retrieval have been described in literature, all of which have their own merits and demerits. Incisions commonly utilised are Pfannenstiel incision and iliac fossa and midline periumbilical incision (Fig. 11.1, Table 11.1).

The extraction incisions are placed prior to retrieval of the graft. The surgeon prepares the incision prior to securing the vessels. It is imperative that the surgeon does not open the peritoneum at this stage. If this is done, this may lead to loss of

Fig. 11.1
Different types of
incisions for
extraction

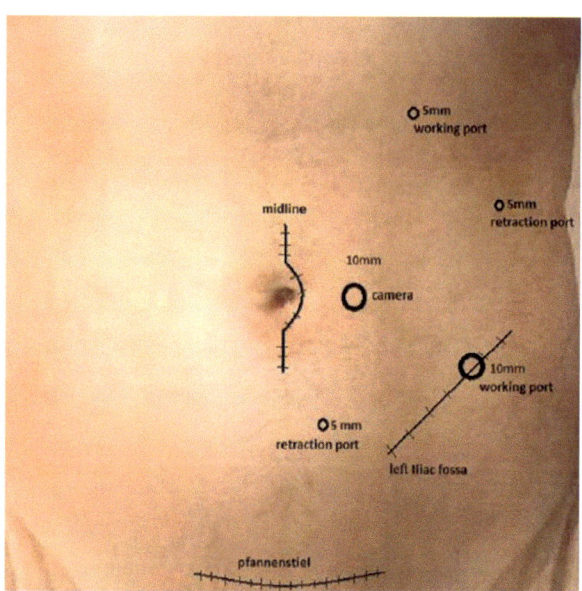

Table 11.1 Comparison between the three commonly used incisions for extraction

Pfannenstiel incision	Midline incision	Iliac fossa incision
Non-muscle cutting	Non-muscle cutting	Muscle cutting
Bowel likely to come in the way	Bowel likely to come in the way	No intervening structure
Difficult to use as hand port	Possible to use as hand port	Difficult to use as hand port
Wound complications less	Slightly more	Higher chance
Superior cosmesis	Inferior cosmesis	Inferior cosmesis
Possible chance of misplacement of the kidney (lost kidney in the abdomen)	Less chance	Minimal chance

pneumoperitoneum and make the procedure challenging. In this chapter, we discuss the various extraction incisions with their merits and demerits.

11.2   Types of Extraction Incisions (Fig. 11.1)

11.2.1 Pfannenstiel Incision (Fig. 11.2)

Pfannenstiel incision is the most widely accepted site of extraction. The incision is widely used in obstetric and gynaecological procedures. The advantages include that the incision is non-muscle cutting and theoretically has less pain. This has potential to reduce wound complications and has superior cosmesis. It may not be safe to extract the kidney through this incision without a hand-assist device, as there is a possibility of misplacing the kidney inside the abdomen with intervening organs like bowel coming in way. In order to avoid this, the surgeon on opening the peritoneum should insert his hand and feel for the grasper holding the kidney. In this way the chance of losing the kidney is minimised. Alternatively, a hand-assist device like Gelport may be used which in turn mandates a slightly larger incision. Comparative studies have proven that Pfannenstiel incision has superior outcome compared to other incisions [7–10].

11.2.2 Midline Periumbilical Incision

Midline periumbilical incision is cosmetic; as most of the incision is concealed under the umbilicus, the incision is typically used in single-port approach. Alternatively, an incision skirting the umbilical skin crease can be taken. The incision offers a more direct approach to the renal fossa. The downside however includes challenges involved in graft retrieval. In case of life-threatening bleeding from the renal fossa

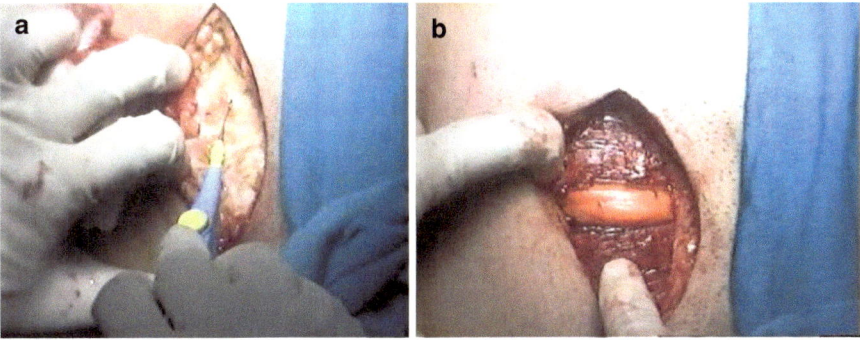

Fig. 11.2 The pfannenstiel incision for extraction. (**a**) The incision being deepened. (**b**) The peritoneum should not be violated prior to extraction as this will result in gas leak

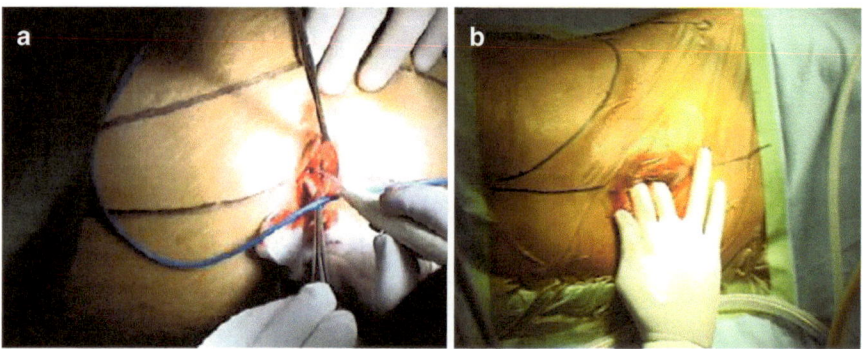

Fig. 11.3 The midline extraction incision. (**a**) The incisioin in the umbilical skin crease is cosmetically superior. (**b**) The fascial incisioin should not be wider than the diameter of the port, if this happens it may result in a gas leak

after extraction, this incision could be converted to a hand-port access. Incidence of wound infection and wound breakdown is more likely because of the tenuous blood supply in the periumbilical area. In obese patients, thick subcutaneous fat and sagging abdomen while in lateral position make it more challenging [7].

This is the incision of choice when employing the single-port approach (Fig. 11.3). The incision is placed at the outset. The single-port device is inserted through the same incision. The graft can be retrieved through the same incision. This step can be made easier by using a Gelpoint™ device.

11.2.3 Iliac Fossa Incision

The kidney can be easily extracted through the incision as there are no intervening structures like the colon. This is the preferred method of extraction in retroperitoneoscopic donor nephrectomy. The muscle-cutting incision is expected to be more painful and prone to wound complications as shown in some studies [7, 8]. This is the incision of choice in obese individuals.

This incision has a direct access to the renal hilum and hence offers a theoretical possibility of fast graft retrieval.

The alternative methods for extraction is using custom made Endobag bag (Ethicon endosurgery, OH, USA), Gelport device (Applied Medical, Rancho Santa Margarita, CA, USA) and manual extraction without any hand assit devices [11]. The retrieval bags offer the advantage of smaller incisions and a possibility of controlled extraction. The drawback of this technique is that the retrieval bags are expensive and cost 500$. With this technique, pneumoperitoneum is not maintained after extraction, and any emergent situation cannot be tackled until the abdomen is closed.

11.2.4 Transvaginal Extraction

Recently few studies have demonstrated the advantage of transvaginal extraction in female donors [12–14]. During a transvaginal extraction, a vaginal swab culture is taken 2 weeks before surgery. The donors are advised to use vaginal pessaries 3 days prior to surgery. The donor nephrectomy is performed with routine steps. The studies have shown that with transvaginal extraction cosmetic outcome and pain score are superior to other methods of extraction [12–14]. Drawback of transvaginal extraction includes alteration in position of the patient and can be performed only in patients with capacious vagina. The authors in one of the series used a modified extractor which helped in maintaining the pneumoperitoneum just prior to extraction. The authors placed the extractor in the posterior fornix; this facilitated the extraction. The authors state that this helped in reducing the warm ischaemia time [14]. Theoretical concern of infection has been the deterring factor in embarking on such a procedure. But till now any of these studies have not demonstrated increased rate infection. [13, 15]. Canes and associates note that this approach was particularly difficult in obese patients. The reasons cited were inability to obtain adequate exposure, poor manoeuvrability of instruments and inability to retract the colon. In addition, difficulty was encountered in placing the patient in modified position. Patients with large fibroids pose challenge as the access through the posterior fornix is precluded.

Kishore et al. in their study note that this approach is better in premenopausal donor with a BMI of less than 31 [14].

11.2.5 Extraction Incision for Single Site Surgeries

Single-incision surgeries have the advantage of avoiding multiple incisions and attendant morbidities of the port site. Various approaches include midline periumbilical and the Pfannenstiel which eventually is utilised as the extraction incision [16, 17]. Various devices used include Gelpoint (Applied Medical, Rancho Santa Margarita, CA, USA) and SILS (Covidien, New Haven, CT, USA) [16, 17]. Dubey et al. have performed this in single-incision multiport manner centred around the umbilicus [18].

The port to be utilised is decided at the beginning. The reason for doing so is that the size of the fascial incision should not exceed the diameter of the probe. If this precaution is not followed, there remains a possibility of leakage of pneumoperitoneum.

The tenets for insertion of ports in such cases are the following:

1. Choose the access port to be inserted before commencement of surgery.
2. Skin incision should be smaller.
3. Fascial incision should be larger.
4. Beware of gas leak.
5. Separate the omentum on the inner aspect of peritoneum before insertion of ports.

11.3   Comparison Between Different Incisions

Kishore et al. in their series have compared three incisions, namely, Pfannenstiel, midline and iliac fossa reduced in Pfannenstiel incision compared to iliac fossa. The parameters compared included warm ischaemia time, length of incision and wound complications. They found that the warm ischaemia time was significantly less in Pfannenstiel incision compared with iliac fossa incision. The length of the incision was less in midline group in comparison to all the three groups. The midline incision group had significantly larger graft extraction complications. The complications included perinephric haematoma due to excessive traction on the fat [8].

11.3.1 Risk Reduction Strategies for Safe Extraction

1. Never open the peritoneum prior to securing the vessels. A rent in the peritoneum causes loss of pneumoperitoneum.
2. The surgeons hand should grasp the grasper holding the graft. This in turn helps in preventing graft loss.
3. The iliac fossa incisions are preferred in obese individuals; Pfannenstiel incisions are cosmetically superior, while umbilical incision helps in single-port approach.
4. The perigraft fat acts as a handle to retrieve the graft. While extracting the graft, the ports should be removed to prevent laceration of the graft.

Conclusion

Extraction is a critical part in laparoscopic donor nephrectomy. It should be dictated by the individual surgeon comfort and experience. The ultimate aim should be safety of the donor and graft and less morbidity to the donor.

References

1. Ratner LE, Ciseck LJ, RG M, et al. Laparoscopic live donor nephrectomy. Transplantation. 1995;60:1047–9.
2. Kieran K, Roberts WW. Laparoscopic donor nephrectomy: an update. Curr Opin Nephrol Hypertens. 2005;14:599–603.
3. Romanelli JR, Kelly JJ, Litwin DE. Hand-assisted laparoscopic surgery in the United States: an overview. Semin Laparosc Surg. 2001;8:96–103.
4. Kocak B, Baker TB, Koffron AJ, et al. Laparoscopic living donor nephrectomy: a single-center sequential experience comparing hand-assisted versus standard technique. Urology. 2007;70:1060–3.
5. Wang GJ, Afaneh C, Aull M, et al. Laparoendoscopic single site live donor nephrectomy: single institution report of initial 100 cases. J Urol. 2011;186:2333–7.
6. Siqueira Jr TM, Mitre AI, FA S, et al. A cost-effective technique for pure laparoscopic live donor nephrectomy. Int Braz J Urol. 2006;32:23–8.

7. Gupta M, Singh P, Dubey D, et al. A comparison of kidney retrieval incisions in laparoscopic transperitoneal donor nephrectomy. Urol Int. 2008;81:296–300.
8. Kishore TA, Tarun BK, Shetty A, et al. Comparison of three different techniques of extraction in Laparoscopic donor nephrectomy. Indian J Urol. 2013;29(3):184–7.
9. Amer T, Biju RD, Hutton R, et al. Laparoscopic nephrectomy – Pfannenstiel or expanded port site specimen extraction: a systematic review and meta-analysis. Cent Eur J Urol. 2015;68(3):322–9.
10. Tisdale BE, Kapoor A, Hussain A, et al. Intact specimen extraction in laparoscopic nephrectomy procedures: Pfannenstiel versus expanded port site incisions. Urology. 2007;69:241–4.
11. Su LM, Ratner LE, Montgomery RA, et al. Laparoscopic live donor nephrectomy: trends in donor and recipient morbidity following 381 consecutive cases. Ann Surg. 2004;240:358–63.
12. Alcaraz A, Peri L, Molina A, et al. Feasibility of transvaginal NOTES-assisted laparoscopic nephrectomy. Eur Urol. 2010;57:233–7.
13. Alcaraz A, Musquera M, Peri L, et al. Feasibility of transvaginal natural orifice transluminal endoscopic surgery assisted living donor nephrectomy: is kidney vaginal delivery the approach of the future? Eur Urol. 2011;59(6):1019–25.
14. Kishore TA, Shetty A, Balan T, et al. Laparoscopic donor nephrectomy with transvaginal extraction: initial experience of 30 cases. J Endourol. 2013;27(11):1361–5.
15. Adiyat KT, Shetty A, PK M, et al. Comparison of bacterial contamination between transvaginal-assisted laparoscopic donor nephrectomy and conventional donor nephrectomy. Clin Transpl. 2015;29(2):99–100.
16. Aull MJ, Afaneh C, Charlton M, et al. A randomized, prospective, parallel group study of laparoscopic versus laparoendoscopic single site donor nephrectomy for kidney donation. Am J Transplant. 2014;14(7):1630–7.
17. Andonian S, Herati AS, MA A, et al. Laparoendoscopic single-site pfannenstiel donor nephrectomy. Urology. 2010;75(1):9–12.
18. Dubey D, Shrinivas RP, Srikanth G. Transumbilical laparoendoscopic single-site donor nephrectomy: without the use of a single port access device. Indian J Urol. 2011;27:180–4.

Troubleshooting in Laparoscopic Donor Nephrectomy

René Sotelo Noguera, Raed A. Azhar,
Jorge E. Gomez Meza, and Oscar D. Martin Garzón

Abstract

Surgical complications are related to the learning curve of the surgeon and, in particular, the first 30 surgical cases, in which the rate of major complications reaches 30%. However, this rate decreases to 20% in the first 50 cases and 6% once the surgeon has performed 200–250 cases. It has been noted that surgeons with experience in previous laparoscopic surgery have no such associated rate of complications.

In this chapter, we discuss the complications associated with laproscopic donor nephrectomy. We focus on predisposing factors, risk reduction strategies for these in the pre, peri and postoperative period.

Chronic kidney disease represents not only a worldwide public health problem but a socioeconomic problem as well. It can result in end-stage kidney disease (ESKD), cardiovascular disease (CVD), and premature death. The disease prevalence and the worldwide use of renal replacement therapy are expected to increase considerably in the next 10 years. This increase is believed to be driven by the increases in life expectancy and increasing prevalence of diabetes and hypertension [1].

R.S. Noguera (✉) • J.E.G. Meza • O.D.M. Garzón
Department of Urology, University of Southern California, Los Angeles, USA

Clínica Cooperativa de Colombia, Universidad Cooperativa de Colombia - Facultad de Medicina, Villavicencio, Colombia
e-mail: rene.sotelo@med.usc.edu

R.A. Azhar
Urology Department, King Abdulaziz University, Jeddah, Saudi Arabia

© Springer Nature Singapore Pte Ltd. 2017
M.R. Desai, A.P. Ganpule (eds.), *Laparoscopic Donor Nephrectomy*,
DOI 10.1007/978-981-10-2849-6_12

12.1   Introduction

Renal replacement therapy (RRT), through dialysis or renal transplantation (living or cadaveric donor), is a life-saving but expensive treatment. A live kidney donor offers several advantages including cost-effectiveness, improved graft quality, and recipient quality. Despite these advantages, the shortage of kidney donors remains a major problem because of the potential risk of serious surgical complications from a procedure in which the donor does not gain personal medical benefit. For this reason, it is important to understand the risk factors for complications associated with donor nephrectomy [2]. Surgical complications are common. For living donor nephrectomy (LDN), any complication is devastating, both for the donor and the recipient; thus, the question arises of whether the condition of the recipient should be a factor in justifying a procedure on a healthy patient [3–5]. As the kidney is considered to be a valuable organ, the surgeon must find a way to secure its extraction while minimizing the possibility of failure.

Surgical complications are related to the learning curve of the surgeon and, in particular, the first 30 surgical cases, in which the rate of major complications reaches 30%. However, this rate decreases to 20% in the first 50 cases and 6% once the surgeon has performed 200–250 cases. It has been noted that surgeons with experience in previous laparoscopic surgery have no such associated rate of complications [6].

When discussing complications, it is important to understand how to classify them. Classification standards objectify the results and help develop better studies. The most well-known classification system for surgical complications is the one described by Dindo. This classification was tested in a cohort of 6,336 general surgery patients when a high level of correlation was found between the level classification and the procedure complexity ($p < 0.0001$) as well as the length of hospital stay ($p < 0.0001$). The researchers considered this to be a simple, reproducible, logical, and useful classification.

Another commonly used classification system is that of Clavien, which does not consider specific donor alterations. Based on these classifications, further efforts have been made to generate new and improved ratings that are all-inclusive, if not widely accepted [7, 8].

12.2   Presurgery Factors

During donor assessment, it is important to understand the risk factors for the development of perioperative and postoperative complications. Living donor nephrectomy is a procedure in which healthy donors undergo major surgery and gain no personal benefit.

12.2.1 Obesity

Obesity is a growing problem and has become increasingly common worldwide in recent years. It is a risk factor for diverse pathologies, including cardiovascular pathology, urinary tract lithiasis, and end-stage renal disease. The later is due to an increase in filtration fraction and glomerular filtration rate, which are predictors of renal function loss [2, 9]. Therefore, it is imperative to carefully evaluate these patients regarding their baseline cardiovascular risk as well as their increased risk of long-term kidney disease.

Obesity is also a significant risk factor of complications after abdominal surgery. Heimbach et al. studied 10 of 21 donors with a BMI greater than or equal to 35 and found that these donors had a greater number of minor perioperative complications and longer surgery times than nonobese donors. However, the occurrence of major complications and length of hospital stay were similar between the two groups [10].

The rate of conversion from laparoscopic to open surgery during hand-assisted laparoscopic donor nephrectomy (HALDN) has been shown to be the same for obese and nonobese donors, whereas laparoscopic donor nephrectomy conversion was found to be greater in obese donors [11]. A retrospective study of 5,304 donors showed no difference in mortality, readmission, and rates of repeat surgery between obese and nonobese donors [12].

12.2.2 Previous Abdominal Surgery

Donors with a history of previous surgery have shown a higher rate of intra-abdominal adhesions than those without, with a rate of 85% (55–100%) in those with prior surgery compared with a rate of 52% (2–93%) in donors without prior surgery [13–15]. This has no negative effects on the probability of surgical success and is not a contraindication to a minimally invasive approach.

Intra-abdominal adhesions lead to an increased risk of conversion to open surgery and subsequent increased risk of patient morbidity. Kok et al. demonstrated this in a study of 161 patients; a higher number of conversions were recorded in patients with adhesions (0% in donors free of adhesions vs. 10% in donors with intra-abdominal adhesions, $p = 0.005$) [16].

12.2.3 Cigarette Use

Smoking not only increases the risk of developing cancer but has also been shown to particularly increase the risk of developing kidney cancer by a factor of 1.8 [17]; this is a significant consequence for a live donor patient. Smoking also affects the quality of healing: nonsmokers produce 1.8 times more collagen than smokers. This leads to a higher rate of dehiscence, surgical site infections, incisional hernia, and injury among patients who smoke [18–20].

12.2.4 Age

Kidney donors who are older than 60–70 years present with a higher incidence of concomitant diseases and decreased kidney function for their age. This makes them more susceptible to surgical complications.

Despite these factors, and because of the scarcity of living donors, the selection criteria are becoming increasingly flexible, and older donors are seen more frequently. Several studies have shown that when selecting donor grafts with similar rates of survival, no differences in complication rates are observed, regardless of donor age [21, 22].

Elderly donors must be rigorously assessed before kidney donation because of their lower glomerular filtration rate and higher risk of developing long-term hypertension [23].

12.2.5 High Blood Pressure

Studies suggest that normotensive kidney donors are at an increased risk of developing hypertension. Boudville et al. reported an increase of 5 mmHg in systolic blood pressure in the 5–10 years after a nephrectomy. Systolic blood pressure increase is presumed to be a result of normal aging [23].

These findings, which have also been reported by M. Cherif et al. in a retrospective study of patients including 321 LDN, provide evidence that the increase in blood pressure may be greater and the rise in blood pressure may increase over time. At the 10-year mark, systolic blood pressure was shown to have increased by 13.6 mmHg and diastolic blood pressure by 5.4 mmHg. Being 60 years or older and having a preoperative TFG were both found to be associated with increased pressure or arterial hypertension at follow-up [7]. According to S.A. et al., the most frequent complication of kidney donation was hypertension, occurring in 37.5% of patients; the cohort in their study comprised 21 men and 11 women. Stratification of the hypertension cases resulted in the following distribution: moderate hypertension in three patients with an average of 160/98 mmHg and minimal hypertension in 29 patients with an average of 145/95 mmHg. Of the 32 patients, 16 had a family history of high blood pressure. All of the participants had a normal blood pressure prior to the procedure [4]. However, researchers in other studies have not found this hypertensive effect [24].

Potential hypertensive donors should have their blood pressure under control at the time of surgery and be without related target organ damage. The risk of kidney disease developing in this group is expected to be less than 1 in 100 [25].

12.2.6 Glucose Intolerance

People with impaired glucose tolerance have a higher risk of developing type 2 diabetes; those with a family history of diabetes mellitus have up to a 30% risk of developing type 2 diabetes and those with no family history have up to a 10% risk [26].

Okamoto et al. studied 444 living donors with a mean follow-up of 7 years and found no difference in the development of diabetes mellitus, renal disease, or mortality among donors with glucose intolerance and impaired glucose tolerance [27].

It is considered a contraindication to donate a kidney to a recipient with diabetes mellitus because of a 25–51% risk of the recipient developing long-term diabetic nephropathy [28].

Potential donors with glucose intolerance or a family history of diabetes mellitus must be advised about a possible increase in the risk of developing diabetes mellitus and consequent nephropathy.

12.2.7 Pregnancy

Initial studies reported that there was no difference in the occurrence of pregnancy complications between kidney donors and the general population [29, 30].

However, more recent studies have found higher risks associated with pregnancy following donor nephrectomy. A study of 326 women, with a total of 726 pregnancies and 106 pregnancies post-donation, reported an increase in the incidence of preeclampsia following nephrectomy; the incidence was 5.7% in donors and 2.6% in non-donors, $p = 0.03$. However, the rate of preeclampsia in the nephrectomy group was still within the range observed in the normal population. The rate of pregnancies with stillborn infants increased from 1.1% in the control subjects to 2.8% after donor nephrectomy ($p = 0.17$) [31].

Ibrahim et al. found that pregnancy after kidney donation was significantly less likely to result in delivery at term (73.7% vs. 84.6%, $p < 0.001$) and more likely to result in fetal loss compared to complications during pregnancy in non-donors (19.2% vs. 11.3%, $p < 0.001$). Pregnancy after kidney donation was also associated with an increased risk of gestational diabetes, gestational hypertension, proteinuria, and preeclampsia [32].

12.2.8 Multiple Vasculature

In 12–33% of kidney donors, multiple renal arteries are present, and in 5–10%, multiple renal veins are found [33, 34]. Multiple vasculature of a donor kidney can cause an increase in the risk of complications in recipients, such as delayed graft function [35, 36].

Risks of vascular complications, hypertension, proteinuria, and Glomerular Filtration Rate (GFR) increase with multiple vessels vs. a single vessel have not been found in recent studies [37, 38].

12.2.9 Anatomic Evaluation

There is ongoing debate about whether donating a left or right kidney is the best option, given the small differences in the anatomy of each. The right kidney is easier to surgically remove, and right nephrectomy decreases the risk of laceration of the spleen; however, right nephrectomy is also associated with a shorter renal vein and an increased risk of thrombosis [39].

Left donor nephrectomy, on the other hand, is advantageous during surgery because the renal vein is long; however, the left kidney is also more difficult to recover. The anatomic location and the proximity to the cisterna chyli cause an increased risk of chylous leak; this risk is nearly 4% and is exclusively related to nephrectomy of the left side [40].

There is no documented difference in length of hospital stay, quality of life, rate of recipient complications, or survival of the graft in right- or left-sided kidney donation; there has been, however, a reported difference in speed of recovery, with the right side being faster than the left [41].

In summary, researchers agree that right-sided kidney donation is preferable because of the faster recovery period and ease of surgical removal [2].

12.3   Peri-Surgery Factors

Traditional open surgery has been replaced by minimally invasive surgery since it was introduced in 1995 [42]. The advantages of minimally invasive surgery include lower donor morbidity, a significant reduction in hospital stay, and improved donor recovery. It is also, however, associated with an increase in cost and operative time. Currently there is a gold-standard technique. Laparoscopic techniques, including laparoscopy and hand-assisted laparoscopy (introduced in 1998), aim to combine the advantages of laparoscopic technique with open surgery. These techniques facilitate a quick removal of the kidney and employ tactile feedback to decrease organ traction and reduce ischemia. The robotic technique has been associated with fewer complications and has the advantages of ergonomic 3D vision and use of a robotic platform [43].

12.3.1 Laparoscopic Complications

Laparoscopic complications are frequent. A prospective study of the Norwegian donor registry and hospital records from the United States identified a range of 6.3% for major complications and of 18–22% for minor complications [44]. The reported complication rates varied; the United States reported a rate between 2.8% and 6.8% for perioperative complications and between 10.3% and 17.1% for postoperative complications.

The probability of presenting perioperative complications increased by 1% for each 1-year increase in donor age (OR = 1.01, $p < 0.0001$). Women were 14% less likely to experience any complication perioperatively after donation (OR = 0.86, $p = 0.001$). Obese donors were 55% more likely to experience the most serious perioperative complications. Genitourinary, hematological, and psychiatric pathologies have all been associated with an increased risk of perioperative complications and are the most serious complications (Clavien ≥3) [43].

One study estimated the mortality rate to be between 0.02% and 0.03%, with pulmonary embolism being the most frequent cause [4]. Risk factors associated with mortality include male sex, African ethnicity, and high blood pressure [8]. The greatest risks associated with live donor nephrectomy are perioperative morbidity and mortality.

12.3.2 Complications of Access

The first step in laparoscopic surgery is to establish access to the pneumoperitoneum. This is the most critical and challenging phase, during which more than 50% of the total laparoscopic complications occur. Mortality rates range from 0.05% to 0.2%, according to published studies [45, 46]. Complications related to access, including vascular injury, retroperitoneal and intestinal perforation, hernia, wound infection, hematoma, and abdominal wall metastasis of the trocar site, are uncommon but can result in significant morbidity and even death [47]. Vascular injury, defined as a lesion of the large vessels, is the most serious complication and occurs most frequently when entering the abdominal cavity [48, 49]. Although the incidence of vascular injury in laparoscopic procedures is as low as 0.05–0.26%, it can cause severe morbidity and death in 8–17% of patients [50, 51]. Researchers believe that the true incidence is greater than this rate suggests [52, 53].

Various technologies and techniques for laparoscopic access have been introduced to reduce complications. The closed techniques using a Veress needle, open Hasson technique, and low vision direct input method have all been used. Although there have been several reports on major vascular injury occurring during the closed input technique, no consensus on the methodological superiority of a technique has been reached due to insufficient evidence. Based on previous studies [54, 55], the Veress needle is the most popular method used by gynecologists; however, novice surgeons prefer the open technique [48].

12.3.3 Vascular Complications

Vascular complications are reported to be the main complications to occur from the beginning of surgery to after the surgery has been completed. They have been reported in 0.03–2.7% [56] of intraoperative complications and may account for as much as 40% of all complications in laparoscopic surgery [57].

Major vascular injury, is the most serious and dreaded complication and occurs most frequently during entrance into the abdominal cavity [48, 49]. Although the incidence of vascular injury in laparoscopic procedures is relatively low, it can cause severe morbidity and death in 8–17% of patients as described above [50, 51]. However, the true incidence is believed to be underestimated by this rate as previously stated [52, 53]. As described above, various technologies and techniques for laparoscopic access, including the closed technique with Veress needle, open Hasson technique, and entry under direct vision method, have been introduced to reduce the occurrence of complications. Although there have been several reports on major vascular injury during the closed technique, there is still no consensus as to the superiority of one method over the others [54, 55].

Additional procedures that can cause vascular complications are radical prostatectomy and either partial or simple radical nephrectomy [57].

12.3.4 Stapler Failure Complications

One study has determined that the mortality rate of donor kidneys 90 days after surgery is 0.03%, with ensuring the patency of both the renal artery and renal vein being one of the most challenging tasks [58]. Vascular control can be achieved through either non-transfixion or transfixion techniques. Techniques of non-transfixion ensure closure by suturing simple loops or clips around the vessels but not through them. Transfixion techniques, on the other hand, bind the suture material through the wall of the vessel, thereby ensuring that the staple or suture material penetrates the artery or vein [59].

In 2006, a survey by the American Society of Transplant Surgeons revealed a significant number of fatal bleeding events in live donor nephrectomies (LDN) related to the inadequacy of certain clips. This discovery led to the contraindication of the Weck® Hem-o-lok® clip for control of the renal artery during LDN [58].

Simforosh et al. conducted a study on renal artery placement of Hem-o-lok clips that were both 10 mm and 12 mm larger than titan clips; they found no evidence of bleeding or mobilization of the Hem-o-lok. Consequently, this was then considered a safe surgical technique [8].

This result led to the wide use of the stapler system, which despite being better and more widely used still has the potential for failure. Failure is defined as instant device malfunction with the inability to meet performance expectations. This excludes issues such as clip size or clip length, patient bleeding, vascular leakage, and tissue thickness. There are few publications that reflect the failure of staplers in urology [60, 61].

The incidence of failures in the MAUDE (Manufacturer and User Facility Device Experience) database is 0.003%. Other publications report faults of 0.2% and 1.7% in laparoscopic nephrectomies. The overall incidence of failures is low. The actual incidence is believed to be difficult to assess, as voluntary reports significantly underestimate the true incidence [61, 62].

Stapler faults include several types of failure: poor staple line formation, incomplete vascular closure between staples, device failure, tissue failure, firing and opening failure, and stapler misloading [63]. In total, 76% of nail failures involve poor line formation and shooting failure, and 47% require conversion [63, 64].

12.3.5 Digestive System Complications

Digestive system complications have the second or third highest rate of frequency of all complications in laparoscopic surgery, with a rate ranging from 0% to 0.9% [57]. Some studies have reported them as being the primary complication [43]. Intestinal lesions, in particular, are potentially fatal if not recognized during surgery and may potentially cause acute abdominal sepsis.

Intestinal injury can occur at any time during surgery. From 1993 to 1996, 639 complications related to trocars were reported to the FDA (Food and Drug Administration). Researchers found that 134 (21%) were intestinal lesions [65]. Of these, six (4.5%)

were recognized and one resulted in death. Ideally, intestinal lesions should be recognized at the time of surgery and repaired immediately by using a technical intracorporeal technique.

A meta-analysis found that the incidence of gastrointestinal injury during laparoscopy was 0.13% [66]. The small intestine was the organ most commonly injured, and the most frequent cause was trocar or Veress needle insertion (41.8%). The second most common cause of intraoperative intestinal lesion was electrocautery (25.6%). Injuries related to thermal damage to the bowel were not reported.

12.3.6 Urinary System Complications

As with digestive system complications, urinary tract lesions have been reported to be the second or third most common complication in laparoscopic surgery, although the incidence in the urinary tract is low, occurring in less than 1% of patients [57]. A review of non-urological procedures reported rates of ureteral injury of 0.09–14% [67].

Regardless of the procedure performed, identifying lesions during surgery can reduce future patient morbidity.

The repair of ureteral injury depends on the specific location of the lesion (proximal, middle, or distal ureter), the cause of the injury (electrocautery, crushing, ligation, or transection), and the length of the ureteral loss.

Proximal and middle ureter injuries are handled with ureteral release, followed by debridement of devitalized tissue, blunting of edges, and closure with continued or separate points. Distal lesions require reimplantation of the ureters into the bladder. In select cases, distal reconstruction is performed, such as with the Boari flap technique or in psoas muscle bladder suspension.

Bladder lesion is a rare event during urologic surgery, with an incidence of 0.7% [57]. It is more common in laparoscopic gynecologic surgery and is especially prevalent in patients with a history of Cesarean section or malignant pelvic tumors [68]. The bladder can be repaired in two layers with absorbable sutures.

12.3.7 Solid-Organ Complications

Liver and spleen injuries represent less than 1% of all complications. The lesions occur mainly in the upper tract during radical nephrectomy, partial nephrectomy, or simple nephrectomy.

When performing right-sided approaches, injuries can occur to the right adrenal gland, liver, and duodenum. The majority of liver lesions can be managed with coagulation, either by administering argon or by combining biological surgical glue and Surgicel. Duodenal injuries require rapid recognition and repair.

Spleen and pancreatic lesions may occur as a result of left-sided surgery. Pancreatic lesions, when extensive, can be managed with distal pancreatectomy. Another option is to use fibrin combined with Surgicel. If diagnosed after surgery, drainage of the collection is mandatory. Any aspirated fluid should be sent for laboratory analysis to confirm the pancreas as the source of the drainage. Persistent drainage can be managed with the administration of somatostatin.

Lesions of the spleen can be managed in a manner similar to that of liver lacerations. In the presence of a large splenic lesion, splenectomy may be necessary. On many occasions, support from a general surgeon is appropriate [69].

12.3.8 Abdominal Wall Complications

Incisional hernias represent less than 1% of perioperative events [57], but a systematic review has reported postoperative rates of up to 5.2%. A total of 96% of these events occurred at sites 10 mm away from the trocar [70]. This rate is important because of the potential impact of hernias on future patient morbidity.

Predisposing factors for postoperative incisional hernia include surgical and technical factors and patient factors. Surgical and technical factors include the size of the fascial incision (as determined by the trocar size and the use of blades versus blade-free trocars), the duration of surgery, the location of the ports (medium versus paramedian), an excessive manual stretch of the fascial layers, the recovery specimens, trocar angle, and the postsurgical closure of the fascia. Patient factors include obesity, factors causing high intra-abdominal pressure (chronic constipation and cough), and conditions affecting wound healing (infection of the wound, diabetes mellitus, chemotherapy, smoking, and malnutrition).

A meta-analysis compared the rate of complications between hand-assisted transperitoneal donor nephrectomy and "pure" LDN. This analysis documented a higher rate of wound complications from hand-assisted nephrectomy (2.2% vs. 0.5%, $p = 0.02$) [71].

A large retrospective study ($n > 5,000$ patients) showed a greater frequency of incisional hernia repair for HALDN procedures than for LDN procedures (0.5% vs. 0.03%, $p = 0.001$) [72]. Natural orifice transluminal endoscopic surgery (NOTES) has been associated with rare vaginal complications, but wound evisceration and dehiscence have been reported.

Removal of the kidney is performed by the expansion of a port, either with a Pfannenstiel incision or vaginally. This process, when performed with poor technical skill, can cause graft injury.

12.3.9 Respiratory Complications

Donor nephrectomy is considered surgery of the upper part of the abdomen, and several studies have demonstrated that patients undergoing this surgery experience altered respiratory mechanics and decreased pulmonary function [73].

Pulmonary complications are considered to be one of the main etiological factors of prolonged hospital stay and mortality. The incidence rate of postoperative pulmonary complications varies from 9% to 40% depending on the diagnostic criteria used [74].

Several studies have reported that the major complications are changes in pulmonary function and respiratory muscle strength. The decrease in forced vital capacity (FVC) of 40–50%, forced expiratory volume in 1 s (FEV1), and respiratory muscle strength can precipitate the development of atelectasis and postoperative pain [74–76].

12.4 Postoperative Factors

The most substantial long-term complication is the risk of terminal renal failure for the donor; this is currently estimated to range from 0.2% to 0.5% [4].

Donors may experience a reduction in the size of their kidney. This is associated with hyperfiltration and a subsequent risk of developing proteinuria and may accelerate the suppression of renal function. In a systematic review and meta-analysis conducted by Gard et al., the researchers concluded that proteinuria in donors was higher than expected in the general population: up to 10% of donors exceeded 300 mg/day. No reports have linked advanced age, female sex, or blood pressure with a higher incidence of proteinuria in the donor. According to the same review, 19.44% of donors had developed a glomerular filtration rate (GFR) of less than 60 mL/min during follow-up [7]. S.A. Azar et al. reported that all patients had normal renal function prior to the procedure and that six (6.9%) showed an average of 1.4 creatinine mg/dL with a high of 1.8 mg/dL. Microalbuminuria has been observed in 10.4% of patients and hematuria in 13.9% [4, 77].

Finally, we observe that renal transplantation by LDN has a low rate of complications. However, surgeons should increase presurgical inclusion criteria to ensure healthy recipients and reduce the rate of occurrence of possible complications.

References

1. Liyanage T, Ninomiya T, Jha V, Neal B, Patrice HM, Okpechi I, et al. Worldwide access to treatment for end-stage kidney disease: systematic review. Lancet. 2015;385(9981):1975–82.
2. Alberts V, Idu MM, Minnee RC. Risk factors for perioperative complications in hand-assisted laparoscopic donor nephrectomy. Prog Transplant. 2014;24(2):192–8.
3. Palace Traboulsi SL, Medawar W, Khauli RB, Abu Dargham R, Abdelnoor AM, MK H. Laparoscopic donor nephrectomy: the Middle East experience. Arab J Urol. 2012;10(1):46–55.
4. Random SA, Nakhjavani MR, Tarzamni MK, et al. Is living kidney donation really safe? Transplant Proc. 2007;39(4):822–3.
5. Reese PP, Boudville, Garg AX. Living kidney donation: outcomes, ethics, and uncertainty. Lancet. 2015;385(9981):2003–13.
6. Duchêne DA, Winfield HN. Laparoscopic donor nephrectomy. Urol Clin N Am. 2008;35(3):415–24. viii
7. Dindo D, Demartines, Clavien PA. Classification of surgical complications: a new proposal with evaluation in a cohort of 6336 patients and results of a survey. Ann Surg. 2004;240(2):205–13.

8. Giessing M. Living donor nephrectomy – the risk for the donor website. Transplant Proc. 2012;44(6):1786–9.
9. Prague M, Hernandez E, Smith JC, et al. Influence of obesity on the appearance of proteinuria and renal insufficiency after unilateral nephrectomy. Kidney Int. 2000;58(5):2111–8.
10. Heimbach JK, Taler SJ, Prieto M, et al. Obesity in living kidney donors: clinical characteristics and outcomes in the way of laparoscopic donor nephrectomy. Am J Transplant Off J Am Soc Transplant Am Soc Transplant Surg. 2005;5(5):1057–64.
11. Gabr AH, Elsayed ER, Gdor, Roberts WW, et al. Obesity and morbid obesity are associated with a greater conversion rate to open surgery for standard but not hand assisted laparoscopic radical nephrectomy. J Urol. 2008;180(6):2357–62. 62 discussions.
12. Reese PP, Feldman HI, Asch DA, Thomasson, Shults J, Bloom RD. Short-term outcomes for obese live kidney donors and their recipients. Transplantation. 2009;88(5):662–71.
13. Ellis H. Internal overhealing: the problem of intraperitoneal adhesions. World J Surg. 1980;4(3):303–6.
14. Karayiannakis AJ, Polychronidis A, Perente S, Botaitis, Simopoulos C. Laparoscopic cholecystectomy in patients with previous upper or lower abdominal surgery. Surg Endosc. 2004;18(1):97–101.
15. Menzies D. Peritoneal adhesions. Incidence, causes, and prevention. Ann Surg. 1992;24(Pt 1):27–45.
16. Kok NF, van der Wal JB, Alwayn IP, Tran KT, IJzermans JN. Laparoscopic kidney donation: the impact of adhesions. Surg Endosc. 2008;22(5):1321–5.
17. Lotan Y, Karam JA, Shariat SF, et al. Renal-cell carcinoma risk estimates based on participants in the prostate, lung, colorectal, and ovarian cancer screening trial and national lung screening trial. Urol Oncol. 2016;34(4):167 e9–16. doi: 10.1016/j.urolonc.2015.10.011.
18. Jørgensen LN, Kallehave F, Christensen E, et al. Less collagen production in smokers. Surgery. 1998;123(4):450–5.
19. Montgomery JS, Johnston 3rd WK, Wolf Jr JS. Wound complications after hand assisted laparoscopic surgery. J Urol. 2005;174(6):2226–30.
20. Silverstein P. Smoking and wound healing. Am J Med. 1992;93(1A):22S–4S.
21. Minnee RC, Bemelman WA, Polle SW, et al. Older living kidney donors: surgical outcome and quality of life. Transplantation. 2008;86(2):251–6.
22. Remuzzi G, Cravedi P, Perna A, et al. Long term outcome of renal transplantation from older donors. N Engl J Med. 2006;354(4):343–52.
23. Boudville N, Prasad GV, Knoll G, et al. Meta-analysis: risk for hypertension in living kidney donors. Ann Intern Med. 2006;145(3):185–96.
24. Ibrahim HN, Foley R, Tan L, et al. Long term consequences of kidney donation. N Engl J Med. 2009;360(5):459–69.
25. Steiner RW, Gert B. A technique for presenting risk and outcome data to potential living kidney transplant donors. Transplantation. 2001;71(8):1056–7.
26. Wareham NJ, Byrne CD, Williams R, et al. Fasting proinsulin concentrations predict the development of type 2 diabetes. Diabetes Care. 1999;22(2):262–70.
27. Okamoto M, Suzuki T, Fujiki, et al. The consequences for live kidney donors with preexisting glucose intolerance without diabetic complication: analysis at a single Japanese center. Transplantation. 2010;89(11):1391–5.
28. Torffvit OR, Agardh CD. The impact of metabolic and blood pressure control on the incidence and progression of nephropathy. A 10-year study of 385 type 2 diabetic patients. J Diabetes Complicat. 2001;15(6):307–13.
29. Wrenshall L, McHugh, Felton P, et al. Pregnancy after donor nephrectomy. Transplantation. 1996;62(12):1934–6.
30. Jones JW, Acton RD, Elick B, Granger DK, Shrub AJ. Pregnancy following kidney donation. Transplant Proc. 1993;25(6):3082.
31. Reisaeter AV, Irgens LM, Roislien J, Henriksen T, Hartmann A. Pregnancy and birth after kidney donation: the Norwegian experience. Am J Transplant Off J Am Soc Transplant Am Soc Transplant Surg. 2009;9(4):820–4.

32. Ibrahim HN, Akkina SK, Leister E, Gillingham K, Cordner G, Guo H, et al. Pregnancy outcomes after kidney donation. Am J Transplant Off J Am Soc Transplant Am Soc Transplant Surg. 2009;9(4):825–34.
33. Belzer FO, Schweizer RT, Kountz SL. Management of multiple vessels in renal transplantation. Transplant Proc. 1972;4(4):639–44.
34. Touches AM, Perloff LJ, Naji, Grossman RA, Barker CF. Living-related donors with bilateral multiple renal arteries. Twenty-year experience. Transplantation. 1989;47(2):397–9.
35. Guerra EE, Didone EC, Zanotelli ML, Model SP, Cantisani GP, Goldani JC, et al. Renal transplants with multiple arteries. Transplant Proc. 1992;24(5):1868.
36. Minnee RC, Bemelman WA, Donselaar-van der Pant KA, Booij J, ter Meulen S, Ten Berge IJ, et al. Risk factors for delayed graft function after hand-assisted laparoscopic donor nephrectomy. Transplant Proc. 2010;42(7):2422–6.
37. Desai MR, Ganpule AP, Gupta R, Thimmegowda M. Outcome of renal transplantation with multiple versus single kidney arteries after laparoscopic live donor nephrectomy: a comparative study. Urology. 2007;69(5):824–7.
38. Rizzari MD, Suszynski TM, Gillingham KJ, Kill AJ, Ibrahim HN. Outcome of living kidney donors left with multiple renal arteries. Clin Transpl. 2012;26(1):E7–11.
39. Mandal AK, Kavoussi LR, Cohen C, Montgomery RA, Ratner U. Should the indications for laparoscopic live donor nephrectomy of the right kidney be the same as for the open procedure? Anomalous left renal vasculature is not a contraindication to left laparoscopic donor nephrectomy. Transplantation. 2001;71(5):660–4.
40. Capocasale E, Iaria M, Vistoli F, Signori S, Mazzoni MP, Dalla Valle R, et al. Incidence, diagnosis, and treatment of chylous leakage after laparoscopic live donor nephrectomy. Transplantation. 2012;93(1):82–6.
41. Minnee RC, Bemelman WA, Maartense Bemelman FJ, Gouma DJ, Idu MM. Left or right hand-assisted donor nephrectomy in kidney? A randomized controlled trial. Transplantation. 2008;85(2):203–8.
42. Ratner, Ciseck LJ, Moore RG, Cigarroa FG, Kaufman HS, Kavoussi LR. Laparoscopic live donor nephrectomy. Transplantation. 1995;60(9):1047–9.
43. Lentine KL, Schnitzler MA, Garg AX, Xiao H, Axelrod D, Tuttle-Newhall JE, et al. Race, Relationship and Renal Diagnoses after living kidney donation. Transplantation. 2015;99(8):1723–9. doi: 10.1097/TP.0000000000000733. PubMed PMID: 25905980.
44. G F, Hear O, Holdaas H, Line PD, Midtvedt K. Morbidity and mortality in 1022 consecutive living donor nephrectomies: benefits of a living donor registry. Transplantation. 2009;88(11):1273–9.
45. Nuzzo G, Giuliante F, Tebala GD, Vellone M, Cavicchioni C. Routine use of open technique in laparoscopic operations. J Am Coll Surg. 1997;184(1):58–62.
46. Jansen FW, Kolkman W, Bakkum EA, deKroon CD, Trimbos-Kemper TC, Trimbos JB. Complications of laparoscopy: an inquiry about closed – versus open-entry technique. Am J Obstet Gynecol. 2004;190(3):634–8.
47. Munro MG. Laparoscopic access: complications, technologies, and techniques. Curr Opin Obstet Gynecol. 2002;14(4):365–74.
48. Dunne N, Booth, Dehn TC. Establishing pneumoperitoneum: Verres or Hasson? The debate continues. Ann R Coll Surg Engl. 2011;93(1):22–4.
49. Makai G, Isaacson K. Complications of gynecologic laparoscopy. Clin Obstet Gynecol. 2009; 52(3):401–11.
50. Azevedo JL, Azevedo OC, Miyahira SA, Miguel GP, Becker OM, Hypolito Jr OH, et al. Your injuries caused by Veress needle insertion for creation of pneumoperitoneum: a systematic literature review. Surg Endosc. 2009;23(7):1428–32.
51. They Mocan MC, Ament C, Random NF. The characteristics and surgical outcomes of medial rectus recessions in serious' ophthalmopathy. J Pediatr Ophthalmol Strabismus. 2007;44(2): 93–100. Quiz 18–9.
52. Chapron CM, Pierre f, Lacroix S, Querleu D, Lansac J, Dubuisson JB. Major vascular injuries during gynecologic laparoscopy. J Am Coll Surg. 1997;185(5):461–5.

53. Opitz I, Gantert W, Giger U, Kocher T, Krähenbühl L. Bleeding remains a major complication during laparoscopic surgery: analysis of the SALTS database. Langenbecks Completo Arch Surg/Deut Ges Chir. 2005;390(2):128–33.
54. Tinelli, Malvasi, Istre O, Keckstein J, Stark M, Mettler L. Abdominal access in gynaecological laparoscopy: a comparison between direct optical and blind closed access by Veress needle. Eur J Obstet Gynecol Reprod Biol. 2010;148(2):191–4.
55. Ahmad G, Duffy JM, Phillips K, Watson A. Laparoscopic entry techniques. Cochrane Database Syst Rev. 2008;2:CD006583.
56. Gill IS, Kavoussi LR, Clayman RV, Ehrlich R, Evans R, Fuchs G, et al. Complications of laparoscopic nephrectomy in 185 patients: a multi-institutional review. J Urol. 1995;154(2_Pt_1):479–83.
57. Permpongkosol S, Link RE, Su LM, Romero FR, Bagga HS, Pavlovich CP, et al. Complications of 2,775 urological laparoscopic procedures: 1993 to 2005. J Urol. 2007;177(2):580–5.
58. Janki S, Verver D, Friedman, Peters TG, Ratner LE, Klop KW, et al. Vascular management during live donor nephrectomy: an online survey among transplant surgeons. Am J Transplant Off J Am Soc Transplant Am Soc Transplant Surg. 2015;15(6):1701–7.
59. Hsi RS, Ojogho ON, Baldwin DD. Analysis of techniques to secure the renal hilum during laparoscopic donor nephrectomy: review of the FDA database. Urology. 2009;74(1):142–7.
60. Deng DY, Stoller ML, Nguyen HT, Bellman GC, Meng MV. Laparoscopic linear cutting stapler failure. Urology. 2002;60(3):415–9. discussion 9–20.
61. Kwazneski 2nd D, Six C, Stahlfeld K. The incidence of laparoscopic stapler malfunction unacknowledged. Surg Endosc. 2013;27(1):86–9.
62. Chan D, Bishoff JT, Ratner L, Kavoussi LR, Jarrett TW. Gastrointestinal endovascular stapler device malfunction during laparoscopic nephrectomy: early recognition and management. J Urol. 2000;164(2):319–21.
63. Brown SL, Woo EK. Surgical stapler-associated fatalities and adverse events reported to the Food and Drug Administration. J Am Coll Surg. 2004;199(3):374–81.
64. Hsi RS, Saint-Élie DT, Zimmerman GJ, Baldwin DD. Mechanisms of hemostàtic failure during laparoscopic nephrectomy: review of Food and Drug Administration database. Urology. 2007;70(5):888–92.
65. Bhoyrul S, Vierra MA, Nezhat CR, et al. Trocar injuries in laparoscopic surgery. J Am Coll Surg. 2001;192(6):677–83.
66. Van der Voort M, Heijnsdijk EA, Gouma DJ. Bowel injury as a complication of laparoscopy. Br J Surg. 2004;91(10):1253–8.
67. Gao JS, Leng JH, Liu ZF, Shen K, Lang JH. Ureteral injury during gynecological laparoscopic surgeries: report of twelve cases. Chin Med Sci J Chung-Kuo Hsueh k' Hsueh Tsa Chih/Chin Acad Med Sci. 2007;22(1):13–6.
68. Boukerrou M, Lambaudie E, Collinet P, et al. History of cesareans is a risk factor in vaginal hysterectomies. Acta Obstet Gynecol Scand. 2003;82(12):1135–9.
69. Lasser MS, Ghavamian R. Surgical complications of laparoscopic urological surgery. Arab J Urol. 2012;10(1):81–8.
70. Helgstrand F, Rosenberg J, Bisgaard T. Trocar site hernia after laparoscopic surgery: a qualitative systematic review. Hernia J Hernia Abdom Wall Surg. 2011;15(2):113–21.
71. Pareek G, Hedican SP, Gee JR, et al. Meta-analysis of the complications of laparoscopic renal surgery: comparison of procedures and techniques. J Urol. 2006;175(4):1208–13.
72. Kill AJ, Bartlett ST, Leichtman AB, et al. Morbidity and mortality after living kidney donation, 1999-2001: survey of United States transplant centers. Am J Transplant Off J Am Soc Transplant Am Soc Transplant Surg. 2003;3(7):830–4.
73. Paisani DM, Fiore Jr JF, Lunardi AC, et al. Preoperative 6-min walking distance does not predict pulmonary complications in upper abdominal surgery. Respirology. 2012;17(6):1013–7.
74. Moraes K, Paisani DM, Pacheco NC, Chiavegato LD. Effects of nephrectomy on respiratory function and quality of life of living donors: a longitudinal study. Braz J Phys Ther. 2015;19(4):264–70.

75. Arozullah AM, Earl MV, Lawrence W. Preoperative evaluation for postoperative pulmonary complications. Med Clin N Am. 2003;87(1):153–73.
76. Grams ST, Schivinski CI, Ono LM, et al. Breathing exercises in upper abdominal surgery: a systematic review and meta-analysis. Braz J Phys Ther. 2012;16(5):345–53.
77. Toyoda M, Yamanaga S, Kawabata C, et al. Long-term safety of living kidney donors aged 60 and older. Transplant Proc. 2014;46(2):318–20.

Open Donor Nephrectomy in the Era of Laparoscopic Donor Nephrectomy

13

Ravindra Sabnis, Abhishek Singh, and Arvind P. Ganpule

Abstract

Open donor nephrectomy has been extensively studied; its safety and utility have been proven time and again. Open donor nephrectomy is a gold standard procedure against which the laparoscopic technique is compared. In the coming pages, we shall try to understand what is the place of open surgical donor nephrectomy in today's world and what are the methods of doing an open donor nephrectomy. This chapter critically evaluates the steps of open donor nephrectomy, including the patient preparation, patient positioning, and instrumentation required. We shall also at the end try to compare open and laparoscopic techniques.

13.1 Introduction

There is an ever-increasing need for living-related renal transplantation. Worldwide out of the stage 5 chronic kidney disease patients, less than 10% receive renal transplant and about 90% die with the disease. The cadaveric kidney donation still accounts for majority of renal transplants in the United States; in the year 2014, 11,570 deceased donor renal transplants were done against 5,537 living-related

R. Sabnis (✉) • A. Singh
Department of Urology, Muljibhai Patel Urological Hospital,
Dr Virendra Desai Road, Nadiad, Gujarat, India
e-mail: rbsabnis@gmail.com

A.P. Ganpule
Division of Laproscopic and Robotic Surgery, Department of Urology, Muljibhai Patel Urological Hospital, Nadiad, Gujarat, India

© Springer Nature Singapore Pte Ltd. 2017
M.R. Desai, A.P. Ganpule (eds.), *Laparoscopic Donor Nephrectomy*,
DOI 10.1007/978-981-10-2849-6_13

163

donor transplants. But in a country like India where the deceased donor program has taken off only in certain parts, living-related kidney transplant is the backbone of the renal transplant program. Living-related kidney transplants have increased in number due to growing awareness, improved safety of the donor, and assurance that the delayed impact of donor nephrectomy would not alter the donor's longevity.

Donor nephrectomy can be done laparoscopically or by an open surgical approach. In the United States, 50% or more of the donor nephrectomies are done laparoscopically [1]. In India, at some centers, all donor nephrectomies are done laparoscopically, many centers are trying to shift to laparoscopic donor nephrectomies, but majority of the centers still do an open surgical donor nephrectomy. Open donor nephrectomy is a gold standard procedure against which the laparoscopic technique is compared [2].

Circumstances where open donor nephrectomy scores over laparoscopy are [1]:

1. Right-sided donor with short renal vein <1.5 cm
2. Extensive prior abdominal surgery
3. If the transplant team feels that laparoscopy would not be safe (e.g., anatomical vascular variations)

13.2 Open Donor Nephrectomy

Open donor nephrectomy has been extensively studied; its safety and utility have been proven time and again.

13.2.1 Donor Selection and Preparation

All donors should undergo a triple-phase helical computed tomography imaging. This would give an anatomical road map to the surgeon. Arterial anatomy is demonstrated in the first phase, venous drainage and parenchymal details are demonstrated in the second phase, and the excretory phase opacifies the pelvicalyceal system. This information help the surgeon plan the side of surgery, and there are no intraoperative surprises. Also a radionuclide renogram is done to establish the differential function. As a rule the better functioning kidney should be left with the donor. The kidney with a surgically favorable anatomy and function comparable to the opposite kidney may be harvested.

A single dose of intravenous antibiotic (second-generation cephalosporin) is administered just prior to induction of anesthesia. One to two litres of crystalloids are also infused prior to induction of anesthesia. A target urine output of 100 cc/h is maintained using crystalloids and mannitol. Intraoperative hydration status can be assessed by looking at the turgor of the kidney and fullness of the renal vein.

13.2.1.1 Instrument Trolley (Fig. 13.1)

Retractors

A. *Self-retaining*:
1. Finochietto chest spreader
2. Balfour's abdominal retractor
3. Multibladed self-retaining retractors (optional)
4. Deaver's retractors (large, medium, and small)
5. Right-angled retractor

B. *Instruments*:
1. Long artery forceps
2. Right-angled dissecting forceps
3. Long Debakey vascular forceps
4. Babcock forceps
5. Allis forceps
6. Vascular clamps: Satinsky clamp, Debakey clamp, Cooley clamp
7. Metallic clip applicator
8. Hem-o-lok clip applicator
9. Rib cutter and periosteal elevator

C. *Ties and clips*: Silk and linen ties, ligaclips (medium and large), Hem-o-lok clips (large)

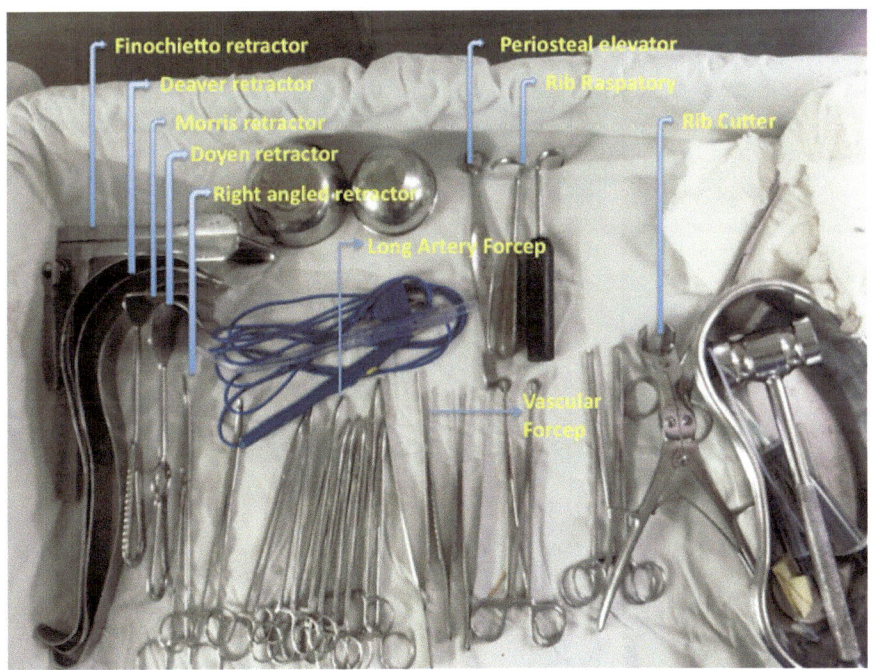

Fig. 13.1 Figure shows the operative instrument trolley

13.2.2 Patient Positioning [3] (Figs. 13.2 and 13.3)

1. Lateral decubitus: operative side up.
2. Flank placed over the kidney bridge.
3. Ipsilateral leg extended and contralateral leg flexed, with a pillow between the two legs.
4. Patient on the ipsilateral edge of the table.
5. Kidney bridge raised.
6. Table flexed.
7. Head end lowered.
8. Patient supported medially with sand bags.
9. Head supported with a ring pillow.
10. Ipsilateral arm rested on a mayo stand and contralateral arm rested on an arm rest.

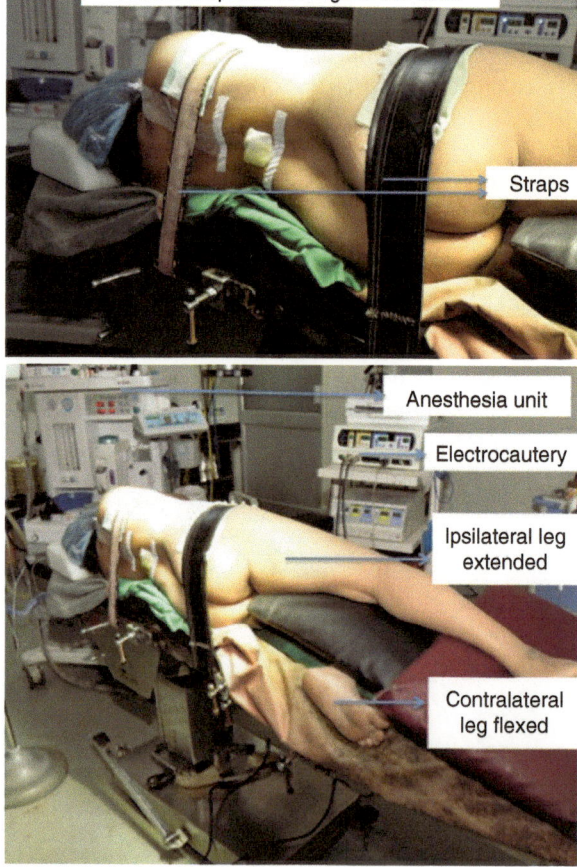

Figs. 13.2 and 13.3 Shows patient positioning

11. Patient strapped at the level of nipples and anterior superior iliac spine.
12. All pressure points are padded.

Anti-embolism stockings should be used in all cases.

13.2.2.1 Surgical Steps

Principles
1. Good exposure
2. Gentle handling of tissue to prevent arterial spasm
3. Preserving the golden triangle of fat
4. Maintaining renal turgidity and diuresis throughout the procedure

Incision [3]
Incision is planned as per the location of hilum on CT angiography. It can be an 11th or 12th rib cutting incision. Incision starts over the rib on the posterior axillary line extending along the rib and then downward and medially in the direction of the umbilicus. The length of the incision will vary according to the habitus of the patient; it can be anywhere between 15 and 20 cm [3].

Skin, subcutaneous layer and the first muscle layer are incised (Figs. 13.4, 13.5 and 13.6). The rib is then encountered, and its periosteum is incised and elevated using a periosteal elevator and then the periosteum is stripped of the rib. After this, the rib is cut using a rib cutter (Fig. 13.7). At the tip of the 11th/12th rib, the retroperitoneum is entered and peritoneum is swept medially. Muscles cut from superficial to deep are serratus posterior superior (posteriorly) and latissimus dorsi followed by external and internal oblique; transversus abdominis is encountered medially (Figs. 13.5 and 13.6, and 13.7).

At this point transversalis fascia is opened, peritoneum swept medially, pleura cranially, and Gerota's fascia identified. Gerota's fascia is opened between two Babcock clamps and perirenal space entered; perirenal fat is separated from the renal capsule, and the kidney is exposed laterally from the upper pole to the lower

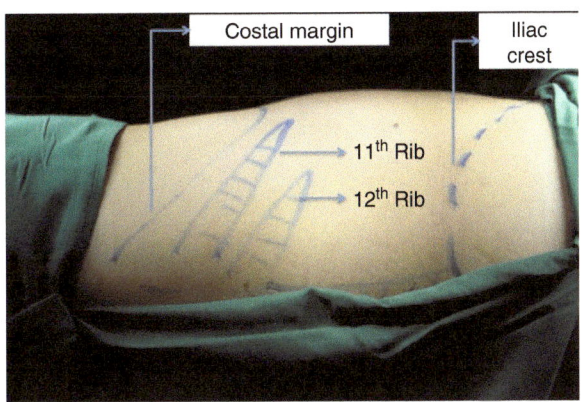

Fig. 13.4 Figure showing surface marking

Figs. 13.5 and
13.6 Figure shows layers
of abdominal wall cut
during the open surgical
donor nephrectomy

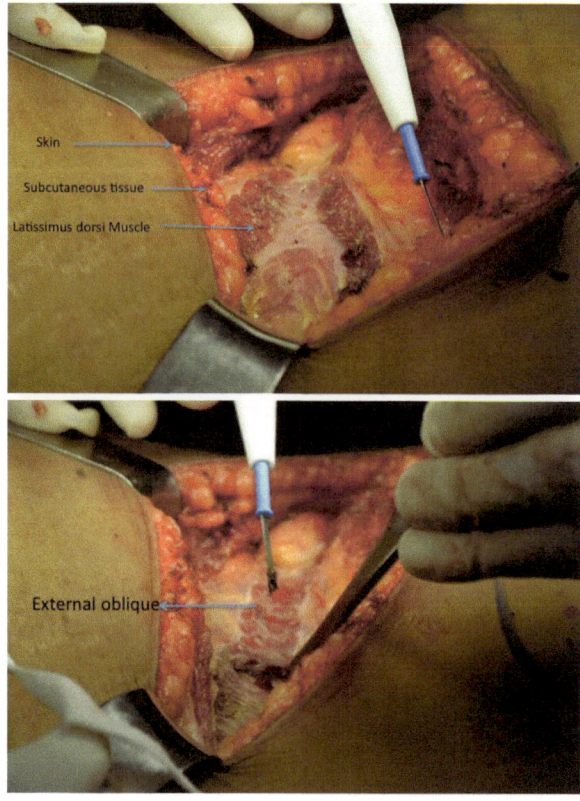

Fig. 13.7 Figure showing
11th rib being cut

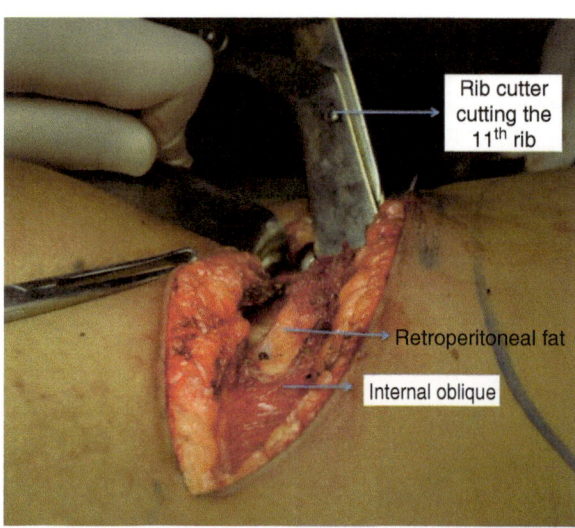

pole; dissection is continued medially taking care not to enter the hilar fat (Fig. 13.8). Now a self-retaining retractor can be placed; it is our practice to use a Finochietto self-retaining chest spreader with two Deaver's retractors to retract the peritoneum and to expose the upper pole. A Balfour's retractor can replace the chest spreader. A single Omni-Tract retractor can accomplish this job [3].

The proceeding after this step is side specific:

13.2.2.2 On the Left Side

The renal vein is identified anteriorly, it appears as a blue hue under perirenal fat, and in obese individuals, the gonadal vein can be identified and traced to the renal vein (Fig. 13.9). Once the gonadal vein is identified, uretero-gonadal packet is lifted en masse and slinged (Fig. 13.9). The adrenal vein is dissected by exposing the upper border of the renal vein; it is then ligated and cut (Figs. 13.10 and 13.11). The renal vein is now dissected circumferentially and toward the aorta till the aorta is clearly visible; in doing so, one may encounter the lumbar veins, which are ligated and cut. The upper pole is now separated from the adrenal gland. The kidney is dissected posteriorly and renal artery pulsations are identified. The renal artery is dissected gently, and the small adrenal artery may be encountered, which is to be ligated. The artery is dissected till its origin from the aorta.

Preserving the golden triangle of fat between the lower pole ureter and gonadal vein completes dissection of the uretero-gonadal packet (Fig. 13.9). The ureter is disconnected at a point where it crosses iliac vessels [3].

13.2.2.3 On the Right Side (Fig. 13.12)

The renal vein is identified and its junction with IVC (Inferior Vena Cava) exposed; IVC is dissected free of tissue for some distance so that Satinsky clamp can be applied on the vena cava. The gonadal vein can be spared on the right side,

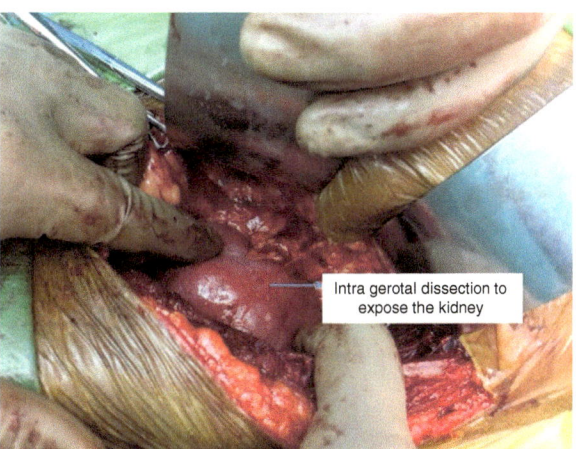

Intra gerotal dissection to expose the kidney

Fig. 13.8 Figure shows intragerotal dissection done to expose the kidney

Fig. 13.9 Figure showing
uretero-gonadal packet
being lifted and the renal
vein dissected

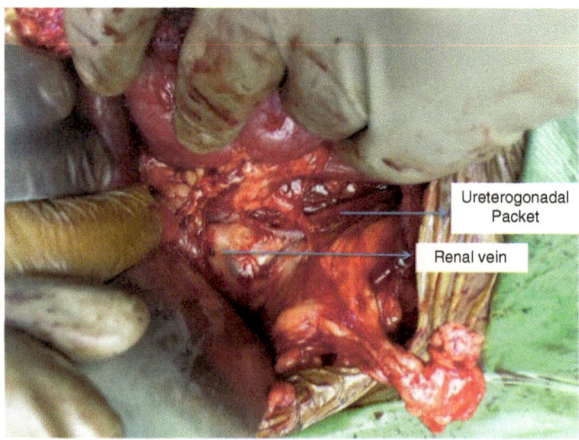

Fig. 13.10 Figure
showing completed
dissection of the renal vein
and ligation of the adrenal
vein

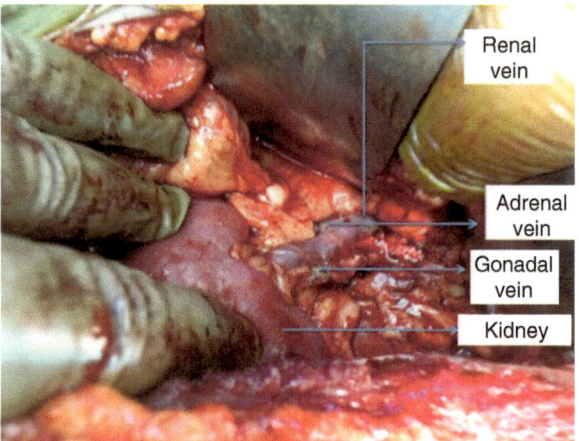

or it has to be ligated and cut separately. Once the renal vein is dissected, the
renal artery is identified and dissected posteriorly and till a retrocaval location.

Retrieval
Before retrieval one should ensure:

1. Brisk diuresis.
2. The kidney is turgid and pink
3. Furosemide and mannitol are given.

   If the above is not satisfactory, one should check blood pressure, check hydration
status, give mannitol, instill papaverine, not handle the kidney, and wait for 15 min
or till the kidney becomes firm and has diuresis. Aminophylline drip can be used in
cases with severe spasm.

Fig. 13.11 Showing completed dissection of the renal vein with ligation of the adrenal and gonadal vein

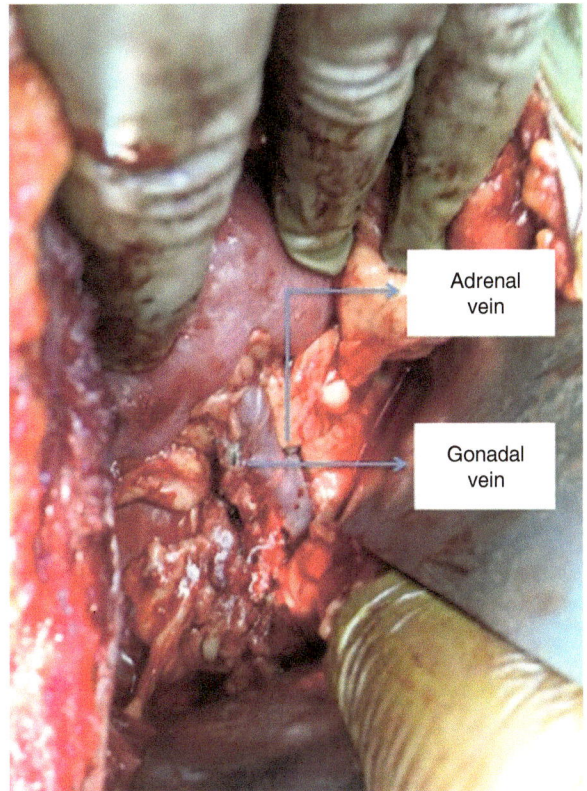

Fig. 13.12 Diagrammatic representation of the right kidney and hilum

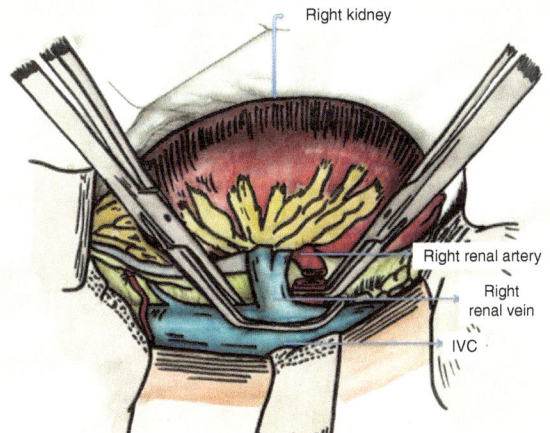

Surgeon should check with assistants and staff that all the things are in place and clamps, ties, and sutures are ready. Some centers give heparin (70 u/kg) on clamping the artery. The artery followed by the vein is clamped, doubly ligated, and then

cut (Fig. 13.13). On the right side after cutting the artery, two Satinsky clamps are placed one above the other, the vein is cut above the second clamp, and the stump is then sutured with 5-0 Prolene (Ethicon, Somerville, New Jersey) in two layers.

The kidney is now flushed with 1 l chilled Ringer's lactate to which heparin (5,000 iu) and hydrocortisone (100 mg) are added. In cases with multiple vessels, largest vessel is to be ligated at the last.

Hemostasis is controlled. Operating field is filled with normal saline to check for pleural leak. If pleural or diaphragmatic tear is present, it is closed over a feeding tube, which is placed in a bowl of saline, while the anesthetist gives positive pressure ventilation. In spite of best of the efforts, sometimes the pleura keeps on tearing, or in cases with large pleural defects, an intercostal tube drain with underwater seal should be inserted. Surgicel™ (Ethicon, Somerville, New Jersey) or Gelfoam is kept over vascular stump. Twenty French abdominal drains are placed. Muscles are closed in two layers with PDS-0, subcutaneous tissue is closed with Vycril 2-0 (Ethicon, Somerville, New Jersey), and skin is closed with nylon 3-0.

13.2.2.4 Pros of Standard Open Donor Nephrectomy [4]

1. It is a retroperitoneal procedure, which most urologist or transplant surgeons are well versed with.
2. There is no peritoneal violation, thus no long-term sequelae of the same.
3. Exposure is excellent.
4. On the right side when length of the renal vein is short, inferior vena caval cuff can be taken.
5. There are almost no concerns of ureteric devascularization.
6. Warm ischemic time is very short; it can be as short as 30 s.
7. Does not require special instrumentation and has short learning curve.
8. Potential side effects of pneumoperitoneum are avoided.

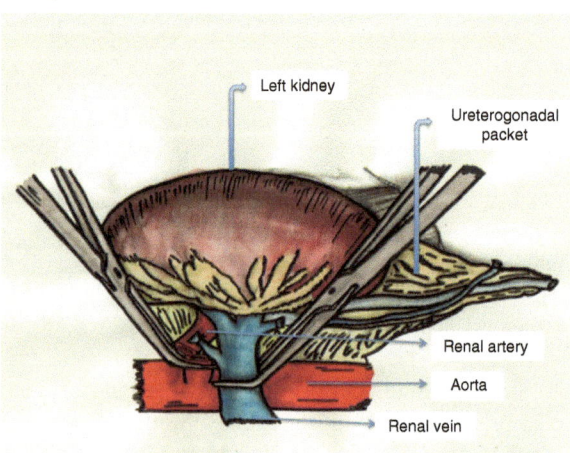

Fig. 13.13 Diagrammatic representation of the left kidney and hilum

13.2.2.5 Cons of Standard Open Donor Nephrectomy [4]
1. Large incision, which is rib cutting
2. Postoperative pain requiring high dose of analgesics
3. Delayed recovery
4. Potential Pleural Injury with its associated morbidity
5. Postoperative paresthesia and probability of incisional hernia
6. Poor cosmesis

13.2.3 Minimally Invasive Open Surgical Nephrectomy (Fig. 13.14)

Minimally invasive open surgical nephrectomy is also known as "mininephrectomy." Shenoy et al. have coined this term and described the procedure [5].

Do no harm is the first surgical lesson that a surgeon learns, and against this very principal is the concept of voluntary kidney donation. So the onus is on the retrieval surgeon to decrease the morbidity and increase the safety of the donor nephrectomy. In the same endeavor, the mininephrectomy procedure was developed.

The proponents of mininephrectomy argue that it is a retroperitoneal minimally invasive procedure; hence, it does not have any long-term problems of peritoneal violation, peritoneal violation like adhesion formation, also they do not require costly instrumentation, and there is no risk of possible graft injury secondary to pneumoperitoneum [5].

13.2.3.1 Principle [5]
1. Incision through which the kidney can be retrieved is used for entire renal mobilization and dissection.
2. Posteriorly a 6–8 cm incision is used to approach the retroperitoneum, as this is the shortest route to renal hilum.

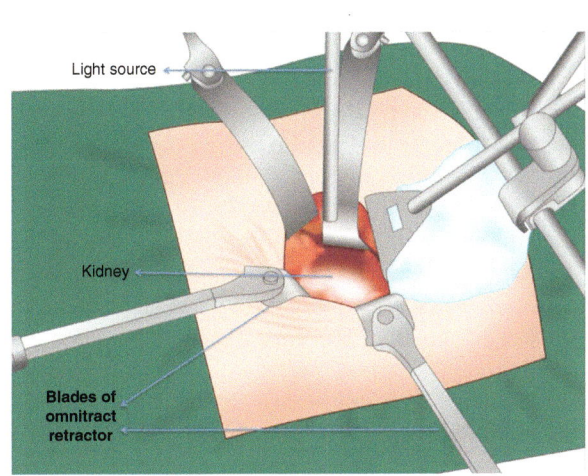

Fig. 13.14 Showing diagrammatic representation of operative field in mininephrectomy. The Omni-Tract retractor blades retract the wound margins exposing the kidney, and then a light source is used to illuminate the operative field in depth

13.2.3.2 Surgical instruments and trolley [5]

In addition to the instruments used for standard donor nephrectomy, the following instruments are used:

1. Multiple bladed self-retaining retractors:
    (a) Wheatlander retractor (Aesculap, Inc., San Francisco, CA)
    (b) Thompson retractor (Thompson surgicals)
    (c) Bookwalter retractor (Bookwalter Inc. Raynham, MA)
    (d) Omni-Tract
2. Operating loupes 2.5×
3. Headlight
4. Long Debakey forceps, ring forceps
5. Long extension tip monopolar cautery

13.2.3.3 Patient Positioning

Patient has to be positioned in the same way as for standard open nephrectomy.

13.2.3.4 Incision

An incision is marked on the 12th rib, 2 cm from lateral edge of sacrospinalis muscle 6–8 cm in length [5]. Muscles are cut to reach the 12th rib; a subperiosteal rib resection is done. Retroperitoneum is entered and peritoneum reflected medially and pleura cranially. A multiple bladed self-retaining retractor is set up to retract the wound.

As the incision is small, exposure is created in parts, using the blades of retractor; only the area of interest is exposed. If the surgeon is operating on the upper pole, two or more blades retract in the cranial direction, and the opposite blades are relatively relaxed so that a skewed exposure is achieved. Deaver's blade is used to retract the kidney and sweetheart retractor blade for peritoneum and pleura.

13.2.3.5 Dissection

Once the retroperitoneum is entered after opening the dorsolumbar fascia, Gerota's fascia is exposed. Gerota's fascia is opened along the convex border of the kidney. The perinephric fat is encountered and striped off the renal capsule and excised starting from the mid pole to the upper pole [5]. This maneuver creates space for further dissection. Retracting the kidney inferiorly, the muscles superiorly, and peritoneum medially using blades of self-retaining retractor upper pole is dissected. Further to this, the kidney is drawn cranially with blades of an atraumatic retractor to expose the lower pole and the uretero-gonadal packet.

The ureter is looped with some periureteric tissue and dissected till just below the iliac vessel crossing. The gonadal vein is dissected and traced to its inversion in the renal vein.

Retracting the kidney downward laterally and peritoneum medially exposes the renal hilum (Fig. 13.15). The adrenal vein is now dissected, clipped, and divided. The renal vein is now dissected completely and lumbar vein clipped and cut.

Following the vein, the renal artery is identified and dissected to origin. All the fibro-fatty, lymphatic, and nervous tissues around the artery are clipped and divided. For the last bit, the kidney is retracted medially, and the remaining areolar tissue is dissected off the kidney.

13.2.3.6 Retrieval (Fig. 13.16)

After heparinization, the ureter is first divided using clips. Hilum is exposed, the renal artery is secured with two large Hem-o-lok clips on a right-angled applicator, and vascular clamp is applied on the renal vein [5]. Vascular clamp can be used on the renal artery also. The artery followed by the vein is cut. The kidney is now free of all attachments; the kidney is now delivered vertically using a ring forceps. The renal artery is clipped if not done earlier, and the renal vein is sutured with 5-0 Polypropylene suture. If the arterial stump is to be tied, a laparoscopic knot pusher should be used, as there is less space for the hand to go in.

13.2.3.7 Closure

Wound is inspected for hemostasis, pleural or peritoneal tear. If any tears are found, they are repaired with 2-0 Vycril (Ethicon, Somerville, New Jersey). Pleural tear should be repaired over a small tube placed in a bowl of saline, with anesthetist giving positive pressure. Intercostal drainage tube may be required on occasions where the complete closure is not possible.

Dorsolumbar fascia and all the muscle layers are approximated individually using Vycril −1 (Ethicon, Somerville,New Jersey). Subcutaneous tissue is closed with Vycril 3-0 (Ethicon, Somerville, New Jersey) and skin with Ethilon 3-0 (Ethicon, Somerville, New Jersey).

In a series of 104 patients published by Shenoy et al., no patient required a blood transfusion. The mean operative time was 150 ± 35 min, average scar length was 6.2 ± 0.5 cm, and length of hospital stay was 2.5 ± 1 day. Two patients had complication and one patient had early graft dysfunction [5].

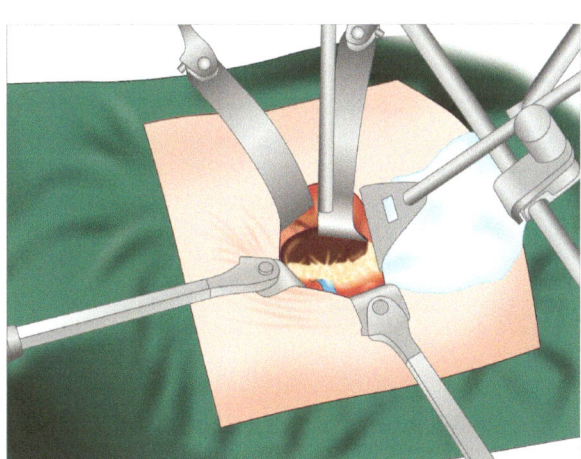

Fig. 13.15 Showing exposed kidney, with dissected hilum in mininephrectomy

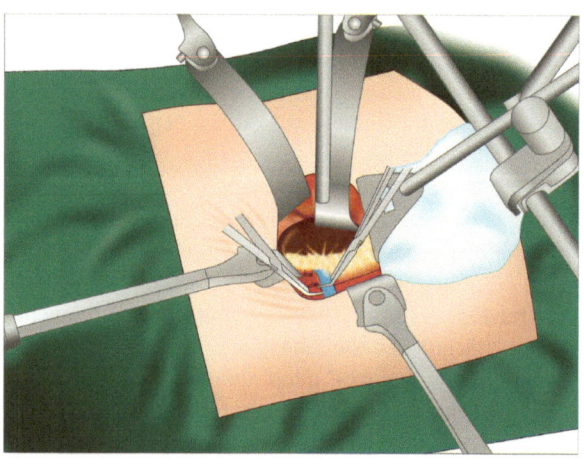

Fig. 13.16 Showing hilum clamped and cut renal artery and clamped renal vein in mininephrectomy

13.2.3.8 Pros for Mininephrectomy

It is an extension of open surgery that has a shorter learning curve as compared to laparoscopic donor nephrectomy and decreases morbidity. It does not require costly instrumentation, and patient can be saved from potential side effects of carboperitoneum; also potentially it saves donor from long-term sequelae of peritoneal violation.

13.2.3.9 Cons for Mininephrectomy

Exposure is critical; at all points in surgery, complete exposure of field is not possible. Continuously throughout the procedure, the kidney is to be retracted using a retractor, and the kidney is eventually delivered using a ring forceps, which might potentially injure the kidney. As oppose to standard open donor nephrectomy or even laparoscopic donor nephrectomy, not many centers have experience with this method, and it has not gained popularity; therefore multicenter long-term data is not available for the surgeons to have confidence in the same.

13.2.4 Intraperitoneal Open Donor Nephrectomy

It is a rarely performed procedure; most common indication in today's world would be an open conversion of transperitoneal laparoscopic donor nephrectomy. Laparoscopic donor nephrectomy is a commonly done procedure; all the donor surgeons should be well versed with intraperitoneal open donor nephrectomy as they may require this skill set in emergency. Another indication would be simultaneous retrieval of any other peritoneal organ like lobe of the liver or tail of the pancreas.

13.2.4.1 Instrumentation Required Remains the Same

Incision
1. Subcostal in case of laparoscopic procedure converted to open
2. Chevron or midline for multi-organ retrieval

13.2.4.2 Surgical Steps

On the right side, peritoneum is incised along the white line of toldt, colon is reflected medially, and duodenum is kocherized. This exposes the kidney, IVC, and renal hilum. The ureter is identified looped, the renal vein exposed, and upper pole dissected; following this, the renal arterial dissection is started. The rest of the dissection proceeds similar to way described earlier.

On the left side, again the peritoneum is incised along the line of Toldt; spleen-renal ligament is cut. The colon is reflected medially along with the spleen. Uretero-gonadal packet is lifted en masse; the gonadal vein is traced to the renal vein. The renal vein is identified dissected, adrenal vein is identified opposite to gonadal vein, and it is then dissected and clipped. The upper pole is freed, keeping the adrenal gland with the donor. The renal artery is identified posteroinferior or posterosuperior to the renal vein and dissected till its origin. The rest of the dissection proceeds as described earlier.

13.2.5 How Does Open Donor Nephrectomy Compare with Laparoscopic Donor Nephrectomy?

Laparoscopic donor nephrectomy (LDN) has evolved, but it is always compared to the gold standard, which is the open donor nephrectomy (OND). When one thinks of the upside of OND, one thinks of decreased operative time and warm ischemic time as compared to LND. Also laparoscopic surgeons have a bias toward the left side; one also thinks about possibility of getting shorter vessels and complication in LND. In the coming paragraphs, we shall see the comparison of the two modalities.

13.2.5.1 Operative Time

One argument for open donor nephrectomy has always been shorter operative time in a study published by ole Øyen et al. The mean operative time for laparoscopic donor nephrectomy (LDN) was 180 (110–295) min as opposed to 140 (95–223) min for open donor nephrectomy (ODN) [6]. Simforoosh et al. have also showed the operative time in OND is significantly less (152.2 vs 270.8 min) [7].

13.2.5.2 Warm Ischemia

Warm ischemic time is less in ODN as compared to LND 1.87 (1–5 min) vs 8.7 (4–17 min) [7]. This has also been proved by another study 1.4 (0.9–3.2 min) vs. 4.3 (2.1–11 min) [6].

13.2.5.3 Hospital Stay and Analgesic Requirement

Hospital stay is decreased in LND as compared to OND (2–3 days vs 4–6 days) [6, 8]. Analgesic requirement in OND is more as compared to LND (36.4{5–98 mg of morphine equivalents} vs 28.1{0–7,798 mg of morphine equivalents}) [7]. The intensity of the pain experienced by patients undergoing OND is more. [7]. The mean time to resume all routine activities is less in LND [10]. Also the mean donor satisfaction is also higher in LND [7].

13.2.5.4 Graft Function

Graft function is comparable in both groups, and increased warm ischemia probably does not impact the graft outcome [7, 9].

13.2.5.5 Complications

The complication rate in both modalities is comparable, but the pattern of complications is different. ODN can cause pneumothorax, flank nerve entrapment, and flank hernia [11], whereas complications with LND include vascular injury, adjacent organ injury, and ureteric ischemia.

After discussing ODN in detail, we would have to agree that LDN is replacing ODN and it is here to stay. But nonetheless all the donor surgeons should be well versed with open technique, as it may be grace saving whenever complication occurs. Also in situations where the renal vein is less than 1.5 cm on the right side and when donor has already undergone multiple surgeries, OND would be the way to do it.

Acknowledgment Dr. Dhanajay Bokare (Consultant Urologist, Care Hospital, Nagpur, India): for providing intraoperative pictures of open donor nephrectomy.

Dr. Ankush Jairath: (Consultant Urologist, Ludhiana, India): for providing intraoperative sketch of the left and right open donor nephrectomies.

References

1. Ahlawat RK, ECAB clinical update: Nephrology: 1st edition: Renal Transplantation, Elsevier India, 2009:43–80.
2. Skrekas G, Papalois VE, Mitsis M, Hakim NS. Laparoscopic Live Donor Nephrectomy: A Step Forward in Kidney Transplantation? JSLS: 2003;7(3):197–206.
3. Cosimi B, Dicken S.C, Open Neprectomy, Kidney transplantation-principles and practice. Elsevier Health Sciences, 6th edition, Eds: Morris P, Knechtle SJ.; 2013:65–70.
4. Barry JM. Laproscopic donor nephrectomy: CON. Transplantation. 2000;70:1546–8.
5. Shenoy S, Lowell JA, Ramachandran V, Jendrisak M. The ideal living donor nephrectomy "mini-nephrectomy" through a posterior transcostal approach. J Am Coll Surg. 2002;194(2):240–6.
6. Øyen O, Andersen MH, Mathisen L, et al. Laparoscopic versus open living-donor nephrectomy: experiences from a prospective, single-center study focusing on donor safety. Transplantation. 2005;79:1236–40.
7. Simforoosh N, Basiri A, Tabibi A, Shakhssalim N, Hosseini Moghaddam SM. Comparison of laparoscopic and open donor nephrectomy: a randomized controlled trial. BJU Int. 2005;95(6):851–5.
8. Lind MY, Ijzermans JN, Bonjer HJ. Open vs laparoscopic donor nephrectomy in renal transplantation. BJU Int. 2002;89:162–8.
9. Brown SL, Biehl TR, Rawlins MC, Hefty TR. Laparoscopic live donor nephrectomy: a comparison with the conventional open approach. J Urol. 2001;165:766–9.
10. Flowers JL, Jacobs S, Cho E, et al. Comparison of open and laparoscopic live donor nephrectomy. Ann Surg. 1997;226:483–90.
11. Jacobs SC, Cho E, Foster C, Liao P, Bartlett ST. Laparoscopic donor nephrectomy: the University of Maryland 6-year experience. J Urol. 2004;171:47–51.